Anatomy
An Examination Companion

For Churchill Livingstone

Commissioning Editor: Laurence Hunter
Project Editors: Barbara Simmons, Janice Urquhart
   Copy Editor: Joanna Smith
Design Direction: Erik Bigland
Project Controller: Kay Hunston
Sales Promotion Executive: Duncan Jones

Anatomy
An Examination Companion

S. Jacob MBBS MS(Anatomy)
Lecturer in Anatomy and Cell Biology,
University of Sheffield;
Member of the Court of Examiners,
Royal College of Surgeons of England

With contributions by
R. C. Samuel BSC (Hons)
Medical Student, University of Manchester

CHURCHILL LIVINGSTONE
EDINBURGH HONG KONG LONDON MADRID MELBOURNE
NEW YORK AND TOKYO 1995

CHURCHILL LIVINGSTONE
Medical Division of Pearson Professional Limited

Distributed in the United States of America by Churchill Livingstone Inc., 650 Avenue of the Americas, New York, N.Y. 10011, and by associated companies, branches and representatives throughout the world.

© Pearson Professional Limited 1995

All rights reserved. No part of this publication may be reproduced, stored in a retrieval system, or transmitted in any form or by any means, electronic, mechanical, photocopying, recording or otherwise, without either the prior permission of the publishers (Churchill Livingstone, Robert Stevenson House, 1–3 Baxter's Place, Leith Walk, Edinburgh EH1 3AF), or a licence permitting restricted copying in the United Kingdom issued by the Copyright Licensing Agency Ltd, 90 Tottenham Court Road, London, W1P 9HE.

First published 1995

ISBN 0 443 04973 4

British Library Cataloguing in Publication Data
A catalogue record for this book is available from the British Library

Library of Congress Cataloging in Publication Data
A Catalog record for this book is available from the Library of Congress

The publisher's policy is to use **paper manufactured from sustainable forests**

Produced by Longman Singapore Publishers (Pte) Ltd.
Printed in Singapore

Contents

Preface   vii

The musculoskeletal system   1
  The vertebral column and rib cage   2
  The thorax, abdomen and pelvis   10
  The pectoral girdle and upper limb   18
  The pelvic girdle and lower limb   30
  The head and neck   46
Picture questions   62
Clinical problems   97

The nervous system   99
Picture questions   134
Clinical problems   161

The digestive system   165
  The mouth and pharynx   166
  The oesophagus and stomach   174
  The pancreas and intestines   180
  The liver and gallbladder   190
  Development of the gut and peritoneal cavity   196
Picture questions   202
Clinical problems   225

The respiratory system   227
Picture questions   242
Clinical problems   255

The cardiovascular system   259
Picture questions   286
Clinical problems   307

The urinary system 313
Picture questions 320
Clinical problems 327

The reproductive system 331
Picture questions 342
Clinical problems 349

The endocrine system 355
Picture questions 362
Clinical problems 369

The lymphatic system 373
Picture questions 380
Clinical problems 387

Preface

Recent reforms in medical education have resulted in a drastic reduction in the time devoted to the formal teaching methods, making gross anatomy a major examination hurdle for many medical students. New medical courses with reduced staff contact time are being designed to produce students capable of self-education. It is hoped that this book is useful in self assessment and revision during an intense anatomy course.

The book consists of nine sections. Each section contains multiple choice questions, illustrations to be labelled, and finally clinical problems. Answers to the questions and explanations and expansions of the answers are also given.

This book is system based. There is an increasing trend in teaching human anatomy in terms of systems rather than regions so that it will fit in better in a multidisciplinary integrated medical course.

Though this book is designed to be used as a companion to the *Textbook of Anatomy* by A. W. Rogers (Churchill Livingstone), the multiple choice questions have been planned in such a way that it can be used in conjunction with any textbook of anatomy. Many of the questions are rigorous enough to be useful also to trainee surgeons who are preparing for postgraduate examinations. It is hoped that in a comprehensive study course in anatomy the proper use of this book will enable the student to build up confidence in the subject.

Sheffield S. J.
1995

The Musculoskeletal System

The Musculoskeletal System

THE VERTEBRAL COLUMN AND RIB CAGE

True/False

1. **Concerning the sternum:**
   a) it consists of three parts
   b) it contains red bone marrow throughout life
   c) the body articulates with the upper seven costal cartilages
   d) the sternal angle (of Louis) is the junction between the body and the manubrium
   e) the sternal angle corresponds to the sixth thoracic vertebra

2. **The sternal angle (of Louis) is a landmark for**
   a) the origin of the main bronchi
   b) counting ribs
   c) the convergence of the pleural sacs
   d) the lower boundary of the superior mediastinum
   e) the thoracic duct crossing from the right to the left side in front of the oesophagus

3. **Concerning the vertebrae:**
   a) there are eight cervical vertebrae
   b) all have spinous processes
   c) all spinous processes are palpable
   d) the spinous process of L3 can be identified on the surface
   e) the pedicles bound the intervertebral foramen

4. **The following statements about the thoracic vertebrae are true:**
   a) all have articular facets for ribs on the body
   b) all have articular facets on the transverse processes
   c) the ligamentum flavum connects the laminae
   d) the vertebral foramen is relatively small
   e) their superior articular processes have anteriorly directed articular surfaces

The Musculoskeletal System

THE VERTEBRAL COLUMN AND RIB CAGE

1. a) **TRUE** From above downwards they are the manubrium sterni, body and xiphoid process.
    b) **TRUE** It is a site for aspiration of bone marrow.
    c) **FALSE** The first costal cartilage articulates with the manubrium, the second to seventh with the body.
    d) **TRUE** It is an important landmark in surface anatomy.
    e) **FALSE** It corresponds to the lower border of the fourth thoracic vertebra.

2. a) **TRUE** The carina is seen at the angle between the two bronchi.
    b) **TRUE** The second ribs lie at the level of the sternal angle.
    c) **TRUE**
    d) **TRUE** The upper boundary of the superior mediastinum is the thoracic inlet.
    e) **FALSE**

3. a) **FALSE** There are 7 cervical, 12 thoracic and 5 lumbar vertebrae.
    b) **FALSE** The atlas (first cervical vertebra) does not have a spine.
    c) **FALSE** The spinous processes of the cervical vertebrae, except that of the seventh, are not palpable.
    d) **TRUE** The highest point of the iliac crest corresponds to the gap between the L3 and L4 spines.
    e) **TRUE** The intervertebral foramen is bounded above and below by the pedicles, in front by the bodies of the vertebrae and the intervertebral disc, and behind by the joint between the articular processes.

4. a) **TRUE** The head of the rib articulates with the body of the vertebra.
    b) **FALSE** The eleventh and twelfth ribs do not articulate with the transverse processes of the corresponding thoracic vertebrae.
    c) **TRUE** The ligamentum flavum connects the laminae of all the vertebrae.
    d) **TRUE** The spinal cord is not as large in the thoracic region as in the cervical region.
    e) **FALSE** The articular facets face superiorly and posteriorly.

The Musculoskeletal System

5. **The body of the fourth thoracic vertebra**
   a) is entirely composed of compact bone ___
   b) is firmly attached to the anterior longitudinal ligament ___
   c) has only one articular facet for the head of a rib ___
   d) has hyaline cartilage on its upper and lower surfaces ___
   e) has its lower border at the level of the sternal angle ___

6. **With regard to the cervical vertebrae:**
   a) all except the seventh have a foramen on the transverse process ___
   b) the seventh has the longest spinous process ___
   c) the vertebral canal is smaller than the vertebral body ___
   d) the trachea starts at the level of the sixth ___
   e) the first thoracic nerve comes out below the pedicle of the seventh ___

7. **The following statements about the atlas and the axis are true:**
   a) the joint between the two allows rotation of the head ___
   b) the axis does not possess a body ___
   c) the membrana tectoria is a continuation of the anterior longitudinal ligament ___
   d) the cruciate ligament lies between the dura mater and the membrana tectoria ___
   e) the ligamentum flavum continues as the posterior atlanto-occipital membrane ___

8. **Regarding the lumbar vertebrae:**
   a) they have short transverse processes ___
   b) the body has large foramina for basivertebral veins ___
   c) they do not allow rotary movements ___
   d) the spinal cord ends at the level of the upper border of the first lumbar vertebra ___
   e) the highest point of the iliac crest is at the level of the gap between the L3 and L4 spines ___

The Musculoskeletal System

5. a) **FALSE** It also has cancellous bone which contains red bone marrow.
   b) **TRUE** But the posterior longitudinal ligament is firmly attached to the intervertebral disc.
   c) **FALSE** There is also a facet on the transverse process for articulation with the tubercle of the rib.
   d) **TRUE** Intervertebral discs are lined by hyaline cartilage. Disc has an annulus fibrosus and a nucleus pulposus.
   e) **TRUE**

6. a) **FALSE** However, the foramen transversarium in the seventh vertebra does not transmit the vertebral artery.
   b) **TRUE** It is easily palpable and is used to identify the other spines in surface marking.
   c) **FALSE** The vertebral canal is larger than the body.
   d) **TRUE** The cricoid cartilage, below which level the trachea and oesophagus begin, is at the level of the sixth cervical vertebra.
   e) **FALSE** The eighth cervical nerve exits at this level. The first exits below the first thoracic vertebra.

7. a) **TRUE** The atlanto-axial joint is between the odontoid process of the axis and the anterior arch of the atlas.
   b) **FALSE** It is the atlas that does not have a body.
   c) **FALSE** It is a continuation of the posterior longitudinal ligament.
   d) **TRUE**
   e) **TRUE**

8. a) **FALSE** The transverse processes are relatively large, the fourth usually being the largest.
   b) **TRUE** These veins are valveless and malignant tumours can metastasise into the bone through them.
   c) **TRUE**
   d) **FALSE** The cord ends at the lower border of L1; the meninges and the cerebrospinal fluid extend further down into the sacral canal.
   e) **TRUE**

5

The Musculoskeletal System

9. **Concerning the sacrum:**
   a) it has five pairs of anterior sacral foraminae transmitting the anterior primary rami of sacral nerves ____
   b) only the upper part transmits the body weight ____
   c) the sacral promontory articulates at the sacro-iliac joint ____
   d) parietal peritoneum covers the whole of the anterior surface ____
   e) the piriformis muscle is attached to the anterior surface ____

10. **With regard to the intervertebral disc:**
    a) fibrocartilage lines the superior and inferior surfaces ____
    b) the posterior longitudinal ligament is firmly attached to it ____
    c) the nucleus pulposus is in the centre ____
    d) the nucleus pulposus usually herniates anteriorly ____
    e) the L5 nerve root passes into the L5–S1 intervertebral foramen ____

11. **The vertebral canal**
    a) does not extend below L1 in the adult ____
    b) contains the anterior longitudinal ligament ____
    c) is bounded postero-laterally by the vertebral laminae ____
    d) contains the lumbar sympathetic ganglia ____
    e) contains the vertebral venous plexus ____

12. **Concerning movements of the vertebral column:**
    a) the abdominal muscles produce forward flexion ____
    b) rotation is maximal in the lumbar region ____
    c) the posterior longitudinal ligament limits extension ____
    d) flexion is limited at the thoracic region ____
    e) extension at the lumbar region may extend the thigh ____

The Musculoskeletal System

9. a) **FALSE** There are only four pairs of foraminae. They transmit the anterior rami of the S1–S4 spinal nerves.
   b) **TRUE** The body weight is transferred to the pelvis via the sacro-iliac joint.
   c) **FALSE** The sacral promontory forms the anterior surface of the upper part of the sacrum; it is the lateral mass that articulates with the ilium.
   d) **FALSE** Peritoneum covers the upper part of the sacrum; the lower part lies in contact with the rectum.
   e) **TRUE** The piriformis originates from the second, third and fourth sacral vertebrae.

10. a) **FALSE** The surfaces are lined with hyaline cartilage.
    b) **TRUE** But the posterior longitudinal ligament is not firmly attached to the vertebral bodies.
    c) **FALSE** The nucleus pulposus is surrounded by the fibrocartilaginous annulus fibrosus and is slightly behind the centre.
    d) **FALSE** It usually herniates posteriorly and may press on the spinal cord or nerve roots.
    e) **TRUE** Each lumbar nerve exits below the corresponding lumbar vertebra.

11. a) **FALSE** The vertebral canal stops at the fused sacral vertebrae.
    b) **FALSE** The anterior longitudinal ligament lies on the anterior surface of the vertebrae.
    c) **TRUE** And is bounded anteriorly by the bodies of the vertebrae, intervertebral discs and the posterior longitudinal ligament.
    d) **FALSE** The sympathetic chain lies outside the vertebral canal, on the bodies of the vertebrae.
    e) **TRUE** The vertebral venous plexus also lies external to the vertebrae.

12. a) **TRUE** The rectus abdominis flexes the vertebral column.
    b) **FALSE** There is no rotation at the lumbar part of the column.
    c) **FALSE** The anterior longitudinal ligament limits extension. The posterior ligament limits flexion.
    d) **TRUE** The ribs limit flexion and extension.
    e) **TRUE** This is especially true when the hip joint cannot extend.

The Musculoskeletal System

13. **The seventh rib**
    a) lies above the seventh intercostal space
    b) articulates posteriorly with the seventh thoracic vertebra only
    c) has a costal cartilage which articulates with the sternum by means of a synovial joint
    d) has a tubercle which articulates with the sixth thoracic vertebra
    e) has a digitation of both serratus anterior and the external oblique attached to it

14. **The first rib**
    a) articulates posteriorly with the first thoracic vertebra only
    b) has scalenus medius attached to the scalene tubercle
    c) has a groove for the subclavian vein behind that for the subclavian artery
    d) (neck) is related to the stellate ganglion
    e) has the suprapleural membrane attached to its inner border

The Musculoskeletal System

13. a) **TRUE**   Each intercostal space lies below the corresponding rib.
    b) **FALSE**   It also articulates with the sixth thoracic vertebra.
    c) **TRUE**   The costal cartilage forms part of the costal margin.
    d) **FALSE**   The tubercle of the rib articulates with the transverse process of the corresponding vertebra.
    e) **TRUE**   Serratus anterior is attached to the upper eight ribs; the external oblique is attached to the lower eight ribs.

14. a) **TRUE**   Unlike most other ribs, the first rib has no articulation with the vertebra above.
    b) **FALSE**   It is scalenus anterior that is attached to the scalene tubercle.
    c) **FALSE**   The subclavian artery lies behind the vein, separated by the scalenus anterior.
    d) **TRUE**   Also to the anterior ramus of the first thoracic nerve and the superior intercostal artery.
    e) **TRUE**   The membrane may prevent excessive expansion of the lung into the neck.

The Musculoskeletal System

 THE THORAX, ABDOMEN AND PELVIS

True/False

15. With regard to the intercostal muscles:
a) the external intercostal muscles are replaced by a membrane anteriorly _____
b) the internal intercostal muscles are replaced by a membrane posteriorly _____
c) the fibres of the internal intercostals are directed downwards and laterally _____
d) the intercostals are supplied by the anterior rami of spinal nerves _____
e) the intercostal nerves and vessels lie between the external and the internal intercostal muscles _____

16. The following statements about the diaphragm are true:
a) it is supplied solely by the phrenic nerves _____
b) the oesophagus passes between the two crura _____
c) the inferior vena cava passes through the right crus _____
d) it moves downwards in inspiration _____
e) the left dome is higher than the right _____

17. The external oblique muscle
a) arises from the lower eight ribs _____
b) interdigitates with the opposite muscle _____
c) has a free posterior border _____
d) has muscle fibres below the umbilicus _____
e) forms the roof of the inguinal canal _____

The Musculoskeletal System

THE THORAX, ABDOMEN AND PELVIS   A

15. a) **TRUE**   The external intercostal muscles extend to the costochondral junction anteriorly.
    b) **TRUE**   The internal intercostals extend to the angles of the ribs posteriorly.
    c) **TRUE**   The fibres lie perpendicular to the fibres of the external intercostals.
    d) **TRUE**   The nerves run in a neurovascular bundle with an intercostal artery and vein.
    e) **FALSE** The neurovascular bundle runs between the internal and innermost intercostal layers of muscle.

16. a) **FALSE** Its motor supply is entirely from the phrenic nerves, but the sensory supply is from both the phrenic and the lower intercostal nerves.
    b) **FALSE** It passes through the left crus surrounded by right crus fibres at the level of T10.
    c) **FALSE** It passes through the central tendon at the level of T8.
    d) **TRUE**   But when paralysed the diaphragm moves upwards.
    e) **FALSE** The right dome is higher and rises up to the level of the nipple (fourth intercostal space) during expiration.

17. a) **TRUE**   The fibres of the external oblique are directed downwards and anteriorly.
    b) **FALSE** The muscle inserts into an aponeurosis lying in the midline anteriorly.
    c) **TRUE**   The internal oblique and transversus muscles do not have a free border as they are attached to the lumbar fascia posteriorly.
    d) **FALSE** Only the external oblique aponeurosis extends to the midline.
    e) **FALSE** The roof of the inguinal canal is formed by fibres of the internal oblique and transversus abdominis.

11

The Musculoskeletal System

18. **The rectus abdominis**
    a) receives a motor nerve supply from the ilioinguinal nerve ___
    b) has tendinous intersections attached to the anterior wall of the sheath ___
    c) has the inferior epigastric artery posterior to it ___
    d) is attached to the seventh and eighth costal cartilages ___
    e) is separated by peritoneum from a full bladder ___

19. **The posterior wall of the rectus sheath**
    a) is deficient at the level of the umbilicus ___
    b) is pierced by the superior epigastric artery ___
    c) is pierced by the inferior epigastric artery ___
    d) is lined by parietal peritoneum ___
    e) below the costal margin contains muscle fibres ___

20. **The lacunar ligament**
    a) is part of the aponeurosis of the internal oblique ___
    b) continues as the pectineal ligament ___
    c) forms part of the floor of the inguinal canal ___
    d) is pierced by the ilioinguinal nerve ___
    e) forms the lateral boundary of the femoral ring ___

The Musculoskeletal System

18. a) **FALSE** The rectus abdominis is innervated solely by the T7–T11 intercostal nerves and the subcostal nerve.
    b) **TRUE** The three intersections lie at the level of the tip of the xiphoid, the umbilicus and halfway between the two.
    c) **TRUE** The artery lies between the rectus abdominis and the posterior layer of the internal oblique aponeurosis.
    d) **FALSE** The muscle is inserted into the fifth, sixth and seventh costal cartilages as well as the xiphoid process.
    e) **FALSE** Only the superior surface of the bladder is covered by peritoneum. As the bladder fills, the peritoneum is separated from the anterior abdominal wall.

19. a) **FALSE** The posterior wall continues to a point midway between the umbilicus and the symphysis pubis.
    b) **FALSE** The superior epigastric artery enters the rectus sheath by passing between fibres of the diaphragm.
    c) **TRUE** The inferior epigastric artery pierces the arcuate line.
    d) **FALSE** The fascia transversalis separates the rectus sheath from the parietal peritoneum.
    e) **FALSE**

20. a) **FALSE** The lacunar ligament is an extension of the medial end of the inguinal ligament. The inguinal ligament is the lower free border of the external oblique aponeurosis.
    b) **TRUE**
    c) **TRUE** The inguinal ligament forms most of the floor of the inguinal canal.
    d) **FALSE** The ilioinguinal nerve leaves the inguinal canal via the superficial inguinal ring.
    e) **FALSE** It forms the medial margin of the femoral ring.

The Musculoskeletal System

21. Concerning the inguinal canal:
 a) the superficial inguinal ring is reinforced posteriorly by the conjoint tendon
 b) the deep inguinal ring is reinforced anteriorly by the fibres of the internal oblique muscle
 c) between the two inguinal rings the posterior wall consists of transversalis fascia only
 d) the inguinal canal is smaller in the female
 e) the inferior epigastric artery is lateral to the deep inguinal ring

22. An indirect hernia
 a) passes through the deep inguinal ring
 b) passes lateral to the inferior epigastric artery
 c) may follow the obliterated processus vaginalis to the scrotum
 d) lies within the coverings of the spermatic cord
 e) may be of congenital origin

23. With regard to the psoas major muscle:
 a) the femoral nerve is an anterior relation
 b) it is a posterior relation of the kidney
 c) it is supplied by the sciatic nerve
 d) its lateral border is closely related to the sympathetic trunk
 e) its lateral border can be seen on X-ray

24. Concerning abdominal incisions:
 a) the linea alba is incised in a midline incision
 b) the anterior wall of the rectus sheath is incised in a midline incision
 c) no major vessels or nerves are involved in a midline incision
 d) the rectus abdominis is pushed laterally in a paramedian incision
 e) in a lumbar incision below the twelfth rib the surgeon may encounter the pleura

The Musculoskeletal System

21. a) **TRUE** The conjoint tendon reinforcing the posterior wall helps to offset the weakness of the anterior wall produced by the superficial ring.
   b) **TRUE** The anterior wall is strong laterally, offsetting the weakness of the posterior wall at this point.
   c) **FALSE** The medial part of the posterior wall is formed by the conjoint tendon as well.
   d) **TRUE** It transmits the round ligament of the uterus which is smaller than the spermatic cord in the male.
   e) **FALSE** The artery is medial to the deep ring.

22. a) **TRUE** And a direct hernia invaginates the posterior wall of the canal.
   b) **TRUE** This is used to identify the type of hernia at operation.
   c) **TRUE** If the tunica vaginalis is not obliterated a congenital hernia can result.
   d) **TRUE** Whereas a direct hernia is separate from the cord.
   e) **TRUE**

23. a) **FALSE** The nerve emerges from the lateral border.
   b) **TRUE** As are quadratus lumborum, transversus abdominis and the diaphragm.
   c) **FALSE** It is supplied by the first three lumbar nerves.
   d) **FALSE** The sympathetic trunk lies along the medial border.
   e) **TRUE**

24. a) **TRUE** The linea alba lies in the midline.
   b) **FALSE** The rectus muscle and its sheath are replaced by the linea alba in the midline. A paramedian incision cuts the rectus sheath.
   c) **TRUE** Only a few small vessels may cross the midline.
   d) **TRUE** If pushed medially, the nerves and vessels which enter the lateral border will be stretched.
   e) **TRUE** The pleura extends to just below the twelfth rib behind the upper pole of the kidney.

The Musculoskeletal System

25. **Levator ani**
    a) originates mainly from the pelvic brim
    b) forms the lateral wall of the ischiorectal fossa
    c) contributes to the longitudinal muscle of the anal canal
    d) is supplied by the ilioinguinal nerve
    e) contracts on coughing

26. **The ischiorectal fossa contains**
    a) the pudendal nerve and artery
    b) the superior rectal artery
    c) the inferior rectal vein
    d) the pararectal lymph nodes
    e) the perineal branch of the fourth sacral nerve

The Musculoskeletal System

25. a) **FALSE** Levator ani originates mainly from the fascia covering the obturator internus muscle.
    b) **FALSE** It forms the medial wall of the ischiorectal fossa.
    c) **TRUE** The puborectalis surrounds the junction of the rectum and anal canal.
    d) **FALSE** Perineal branches of S4 and the pudendal nerve supply levator ani.
    e) **TRUE** It contributes to the rise in intra-abdominal pressure that occurs.

26. a) **TRUE** These structures lie in the pudendal canal on the lateral wall of the ischiorectal fossa.
    b) **FALSE**
    c) **TRUE** The inferior rectal vein runs with the artery and nerve.
    d) **FALSE**
    e) **FALSE**

The Musculoskeletal System

THE PECTORAL GIRDLE AND UPPER LIMB

True/False

27. With regard to the clavicle:
   a) only the lateral end is palpable ____
   b) the coracoclavicular ligament is attached to the conoid tubercle ____
   c) it fractures when one falls on the outstretched hand ____
   d) it commonly fractures in its middle ____
   e) the shoulder usually droops when the clavicle is fractured ____

28. The medial epicondyle of the humerus
   a) is the origin of the common tendon of the muscles of the extensor compartment of the arm ____
   b) lies at the same level as the olecranon when the elbow is flexed ____
   c) lies anterior to the ulnar nerve ____
   d) projects in the same direction as the articular surface of the head of the humerus ____
   e) is more prominent than the lateral epicondyle ____

29. The following muscles insert into the greater tuberosity:
   a) supraspinatus ____
   b) teres minor ____
   c) subscapularis ____
   d) teres major ____
   e) infraspinatus ____

30. The scaphoid bone articulates with
   a) the trapezium ____
   b) the first metacarpal bone ____
   c) the radius ____
   d) the ulna ____
   e) the triquetral ____

The Musculoskeletal System

THE PECTORAL GIRDLE AND UPPER LIMB

27. a) **FALSE** The clavicle is palpable throughout its length.
    b) **TRUE** The coracoclavicular ligament stabilises the coracoid process on the clavicle.
    c) **TRUE** This is because the costoclavicular and coracoclavicular ligaments are stronger than the clavicle.
    d) **TRUE**
    e) **TRUE** The weight of the arm contributes to this displacement.

28. a) **FALSE** The medial epicondyle is the origin of the common tendon for the flexors of the forearm.
    b) **FALSE** Both epicondyles and the olecranon process lie on the same level when the elbow joint is extended.
    c) **TRUE** The ulnar nerve can be damaged here.
    d) **TRUE**
    e) **TRUE**

29. a) **TRUE**
    b) **TRUE**
    c) **FALSE** Subscapularis inserts into the lesser tuberosity.
    d) **FALSE** Teres major inserts into the bicipital groove with latissimus dorsi and pectoralis major.
    e) **TRUE**

30. a) **TRUE**
    b) **FALSE** The trapezium articulates with the first metacarpal distally.
    c) **TRUE**
    d) **FALSE**
    e) **FALSE** This bone is separated from the scaphoid by the lunate.

The Musculoskeletal System

31. **The scaphoid bone**
    a) can fracture due to a fall on the outstretched hand
    b) is commonly fractured in the young
    c) produces tenderness in the anatomical snuffbox when fractured
    d) may receive its blood supply through both its proximal and distal ends
    e) has relatively less periosteum-covered area

32. **Concerning deltoid:**
    a) it has an extensive range of action as it is a multipennate muscle
    b) it flexes and extends the shoulder
    c) it is supplied by the radial nerve
    d) it may be paralysed in a fracture of the surgical neck of the humerus
    e) the skin over the point of insertion of deltoid is supplied by the axillary nerve

33. **With regard to serratus anterior:**
    a) it arises from the lower eight ribs
    b) it inserts into the medial border of the scapula
    c) it acts along with trapezius in abduction of the arm to 180°
    d) its nerve supply is from the thoracodorsal nerve
    e) paralysis leads to winging of the scapula

34. **The following statements about pectoralis major are true:**
    a) it is a lateral rotator of the arm
    b) the sternocostal head is the chief adductor
    c) it forms the anterior wall of the axilla
    d) it is part of the rotator cuff
    e) it is supplied by the axillary nerve

The Musculoskeletal System

31. a) **TRUE**
b) **TRUE** A fractured scaphoid due to a fall on the outstretched hand is most common in young adults.
c) **TRUE** The anatomical snuffbox lies between the tendons of extensor pollicis brevis and extensor pollicis longus at the wrist.
d) **TRUE** Sometimes the blood supply is from the distal end only; this is important if the scaphoid fractures, as the proximal fragment will have no blood supply. Avascular necrosis may then occur.
e) **TRUE** Hence the bone has a poor blood supply.

32. a) **FALSE** The multipennate arrangement gives more power to the muscle.
b) **TRUE** The anterior fibres flex, the posterior fibres extend and the middle fibres abduct the shoulder.
c) **FALSE** The axillary nerve supplies the deltoid.
d) **TRUE** The axillary nerve winds round the surgical neck of the humerus.
e) **TRUE** This area is tested for sensation to rule out axillary nerve injury in shoulder dislocations.

33. a) **FALSE** It originates from the upper eight ribs.
b) **TRUE** On its costal surface.
c) **TRUE** These two muscles produce forward rotation of the scapula.
d) **FALSE** Serratus anterior is supplied by the long thoracic nerve of Bell.
e) **TRUE** The medial border and the inferior angle of the scapula become more prominent.

34. a) **FALSE** Pectoralis major medially rotates the arm.
b) **TRUE** The clavicular head of the muscle flexes the shoulder.
c) **TRUE** The posterior wall is formed by latissimus dorsi, teres major and subscapularis.
d) **FALSE** The rotator cuff muscles are subscapularis, supraspinatus, infraspinatus and teres minor.
e) **FALSE** It is supplied by the medial and lateral pectoral nerves.

The Musculoskeletal System

35. **Concerning the axilla:**
    a) pectoralis minor and major form the lateral wall
    b) it contains the third part of the subclavian artery
    c) it contains the lower trunk of brachial plexus
    d) its medial wall contains the long thoracic nerve of Bell
    e) teres minor forms part of the posterior wall

36. **Concerning flexor digitorum superficialis:**
    a) its actions are entirely mimicked by profundus
    b) it inserts into the margins of the distal phalanges
    c) it is supplied by the median nerve
    d) the median nerve lies under it in the forearm
    e) the lumbricals take origin from it

37. **The lumbricals**
    a) can flex the metacarpophalangeal joints
    b) can flex the interphalangeal joints
    c) are all innervated by the ulnar nerve
    d) can abduct the metacarpophalangeal joints
    e) insert into the dorsal expansion

38. **With regard to the interossei:**
    a) each finger has two of them
    b) the palmar interossei are innervated by the median nerve
    c) the middle finger has two dorsal interossei
    d) the palmar interossei abduct the fingers
    e) together with the lumbricals the interossei can flex the metacarpophalangeal joints while keeping the interphalangeal joints extended

The Musculoskeletal System

35. a) **FALSE** These muscles form the anterior wall. The lateral wall is formed by the upper end of the humerus with the short head of biceps and the coracobrachialis.
   b) **FALSE** The subclavian artery is in the neck. It becomes the axillary artery at the outer border of the first rib.
   c) **FALSE** The trunks of the brachial plexus are in the neck.
   d) **TRUE** This lies on the surface of the serratus anterior and supplies this muscle. The nerve is vulnerable in surgical dissections of the axilla.
   e) **FALSE** Teres major contributes to the posterior wall of the axilla.

36. a) **TRUE**
   b) **FALSE** Flexor digitorum superficialis inserts into the middle phalanx.
   c) **TRUE**
   d) **TRUE** The median nerve lies under superficialis and on top of profundus in the forearm.
   e) **FALSE** The lumbricals originate from the tendons of flexor digitorum profundus.

37. a) **TRUE**
   b) **FALSE** The lumbricals extend the interphalangeal joints.
   c) **FALSE** The lateral two lumbricals are supplied by the median nerve; the medial two lumbricals are supplied by the ulnar nerve.
   d) **FALSE** The dorsal interossei abduct the digits.
   e) **TRUE**

38. a) **FALSE** The thumb and the little finger have only one each.
   b) **FALSE** All the interossei are innervated by the ulnar nerve.
   c) **TRUE** It has no palmar interosseus.
   d) **FALSE** They adduct the fingers.
   e) **TRUE**

The Musculoskeletal System

39. **The following statements concerning the shoulder joint are true:**
    a) the bony surfaces permit a lot of movement
    b) stability of the joint depends mainly on the glenoid labrum
    c) the subscapularis bursa communicates with the synovial cavity
    d) the long head of triceps passes through the synovial cavity
    e) the subacromial bursa lies above the supraspinatus tendon

40. **The following muscles abduct the arm:**
    a) supraspinatus
    b) pectoralis major
    c) deltoid
    d) trapezius
    e) latissimus dorsi

41. **Abduction of the arm to 180°**
    a) requires pectoralis major
    b) requires trapezius
    c) requires lateral rotation of the humerus
    d) is interfered with in dislocation of the shoulder
    e) is interfered with in fracture of the clavicle

42. **In the shoulder region**
    a) the coracoacromial ligament is part of the shoulder joint capsule
    b) the rounded contour of the shoulder is due to the rotator cuff muscles
    c) the axillary nerve encircles the surgical neck of the humerus
    d) cutaneous innervation is by the supraclavicular nerves
    e) the subacromial bursa is prone to inflammation from degenerative disease of the infraspinatus tendon

The Musculoskeletal System

39. a) **TRUE**
b) **FALSE** Stability is maintained by the rotator cuff muscles.
c) **TRUE** It communicates through a gap in the anterior part of the capsule.
d) **FALSE** The long head of biceps is attached to the supraglenoid tubercle within the synovial cavity.
e) **TRUE** The subacromial bursa lies under the coraco-acromial ligament.

40. a) **TRUE**
b) **FALSE** Pectoralis major adducts the arm.
c) **TRUE** Deltoid and supraspinatus abduct the arm up to 90°.
d) **TRUE** Trapezius enables the arm to be abducted above 90°.
e) **FALSE** Latissimus dorsi adducts the arm.

41. a) **FALSE**
b) **TRUE** Trapezius rotates the scapula with serratus anterior.
c) **TRUE** Lateral rotation is performed by teres minor and infraspinatus.
d) **TRUE**
e) **TRUE** Rotation of the scapula is aided by movement of the clavicle.

42. a) **FALSE** The capsule attaches beyond the glenoid labrum on the scapula and the anatomical neck of the humerus except medially, where it is attached to the surgical neck.
b) **FALSE** The deltoid muscle produces the shape of the shoulder.
c) **TRUE** The axillary nerve supplies teres minor and deltoid. The nerve can be injured in dislocation of the shoulder joint.
d) **TRUE** The supraclavicular nerves also supply the skin on the chest as far down as the second rib.
e) **FALSE** Subacromial bursitis is due to degeneration of the supraspinatus tendon.

The Musculoskeletal System

43. **Concerning the elbow joint:**
    a) it has a common synovial cavity with the superior radio-ulnar joint
    b) the normal carrying angle is more pronounced in males.
    c) the ulna articulates with the trochlear surface of the humerus
    d) the articular surfaces are coated with fibrocartilage
    e) it is the primary site of pronation and supination

44. **Carpal tunnel syndrome**
    a) is caused by compression of the ulnar nerve under a tight flexor retinaculum
    b) produces symptoms that include wasting and weakness of the hypothenar muscles
    c) does not prevent the terminal phalanx of the thumb from flexing normally
    d) is also known as Dupuytren's contracture
    e) will interfere with the function of the flexor carpi ulnaris

45. **Dislocation of the shoulder joint**
    a) usually occurs with tearing of the inferior part of the capsule
    b) may damage the axillary nerve
    c) will flatten the contour of the shoulder
    d) will cause the acromion process to be more prominent
    e) usually occurs while falling on the outstretched hand

46. **Muscles important in carrying out pronation are**
    a) biceps
    b) brachialis
    c) pronator quadratus
    d) anconeus
    e) pronator teres

The Musculoskeletal System

43. a) **TRUE**
    b) **FALSE** The carrying angle is greater in females.
    c) **TRUE**
    d) **FALSE** They are covered by hyaline cartilage.
    e) **FALSE** The elbow can only flex and extend. Pronation and supination occur at the radio-ulnar joints.

44. a) **FALSE** It is compression of the median nerve in the carpal tunnel that produces carpal tunnel syndrome.
    b) **FALSE** The thenar muscles will be affected.
    c) **TRUE** Flexion of the interphalangeal joint of the thumb will be possible as this movement is produced by flexor pollicis longus.
    d) **FALSE** Dupuytren's contracture is caused by scarring of the palmar aponeurosis.
    e) **FALSE** The muscle is supplied by the ulnar nerve and it does not go through the carpal tunnel.

45. a) **TRUE** The inferior part of the capsule is the weakest.
    b) **TRUE** The axillary nerve passes through the quadrilateral space inferior to the shoulder joint.
    c) **TRUE** The upper end of the humerus will be misplaced.
    d) **TRUE** This is caused by the displacement of the greater tubercle.
    e) **TRUE** Dislocation inferiorly usually occurs during a fall when the arm is violently abducted.

46. a) **FALSE** Biceps supinates the forearm.
    b) **FALSE** Brachialis flexes the elbow joint.
    c) **TRUE** Pronator quadratus is attached to the distal ends of the radius and ulnar. It is supplied by the anterior interosseus nerve.
    d) **TRUE** Anconeus may cause slight abduction of the ulna during pronation.
    e) **TRUE**

The Musculoskeletal System

47. **Muscles important in carrying out supination are**
    a) triceps
    b) brachioradialis
    c) biceps
    d) supinator
    e) brachialis

48. **With regard to the thenar muscles:**
    a) all are attached to the flexor retinaculum
    b) all are supplied by the radial nerve
    c) abductor pollicis brevis is inserted into the first metacarpal bone
    d) opponens pollicis lies deep to the flexor pollicis brevis
    e) paralysis interferes with the precision grip

49. **The power grip**
    a) may vary in the position of the digits according to the object grasped
    b) is crucially dependent on the long flexor muscles in the forearm
    c) does not require the extensor muscles of the forearm
    d) is affected in wrist drop
    e) is affected in damage of the median nerve at the elbow

The Musculoskeletal System

47. a) **FALSE** Triceps extends the elbow joint.
   b) **FALSE** It flexes the elbow joint in the midprone position. It may have a weak pronating action from the fully supine to midprone position.
   c) **TRUE** It is a powerful supinator.
   d) **TRUE** Supinator is supplied by the radial nerve. It is a weak supinator when the forearm is extended.
   e) **FALSE** It flexes the elbow joint.

48. a) **TRUE**
   b) **FALSE** All are supplied by the median nerve.
   c) **FALSE** It is inserted into the proximal phalanx of the thumb with flexor pollicis brevis.
   d) **TRUE**
   e) **TRUE** Opposition of the thumb by the thenar muscles is essential for the precision grip.

49. a) **TRUE**
   b) **TRUE** They give the power for the grip.
   c) **FALSE** Flexion of the digits is difficult without extension of the wrist.
   d) **TRUE** The wrist remains flexed in wrist drop. It is caused by injury to the radial nerve paralysing the extensors of the wrist.
   e) **TRUE** The flexors of the digits are mostly supplied by the median nerve.

The Musculoskeletal System

THE PELVIC GIRDLE AND LOWER LIMB

True/False

50. **The following structures pass through the greater sciatic foramen:**
    a) the sciatic nerve
    b) the internal pudendal artery
    c) the nerve to quadratus femoris
    d) the posterior femoral cutaneous nerve
    e) the nerve to obturator externus

51. **Concerning the acetabulum:**
    a) only the ilium and ischium contribute to its formation
    b) it is completely lined by hyaline cartilage
    c) the acetabular labrum is made of hyaline cartilage
    d) the acetabular margin forms a complete ring
    e) the transverse acetabular ligament is attached to the head of the femur

52. **The head of the femur**
    a) has an articular surface of more than half a sphere
    b) is wholly intracapsular
    c) transmits the body weight to the lower limb
    d) has a ligament attached to it
    e) receives most of its blood supply through the neck

The Musculoskeletal System

THE PELVIC GIRDLE AND LOWER LIMB

50. a) **TRUE** It passes below the piriformis.
    b) **TRUE** The artery and the pudendal nerve leave the pelvis through the greater sciatic foramen and enter the perineum through the lesser sciatic foramen.
    c) **TRUE** The nerve also supplies the inferior gemellus muscle.
    d) **TRUE** It supplies the back of the thigh and upper part of the back of the leg.
    e) **FALSE** Obturator externus is supplied by the obturator nerve, which passes through the obturator foramen.

51. a) **FALSE** The acetabulum is formed from the ilium, ischium and pubis.
    b) **FALSE** The cartilage forms a horse-shoe shaped covering within the acetabulum.
    c) **FALSE** The labrum consists of fibrocartilage which surrounds the hyaline cartilage.
    d) **TRUE** The transverse ligament crosses the acetabular notch to complete the ring.
    e) **FALSE** The ligament of the head of the femur is attached to the transverse ligament and to the head of femur.

52. a) **TRUE**
    b) **TRUE** The capsule of the joint is attached beyond the acetabular labrum medially and to the neck of the femur laterally.
    c) **TRUE**
    d) **TRUE** The ligament of the head is attached at the fovea.
    e) **TRUE** The vessels lie in the retinacula in the neck.

The Musculoskeletal System

53. **The neck of the femur**
    a) is bounded posteriorly by the intertrochanteric line ____
    b) is wholly intracapsular ____
    c) is closely related to the obturator externus muscle ____
    d) may lead to avascular necrosis of the head when fractured ____
    e) causes medial rotation of the thigh when fractured ____

54. **The patella**
    a) may be considered as a sesamoid bone ____
    b) is stabilised against lateral displacement by greater prominence of the lateral femoral condyle ____
    c) gives attachment to fibres of the vastus medialis muscle ____
    d) has a larger medial articular surface as compared to lateral articular surface ____
    e) has its articular surface lined by synovial membrane ____

55. **Which structures are closely related to the lower end of the femur?**
    a) popliteal vein ____
    b) tibial nerve ____
    c) popliteal artery ____
    d) common peroneal nerve ____
    e) suprapatellar bursa ____

56. **The following muscles are attached to the fibula:**
    a) extensor digitorum longus ____
    b) flexor digitorum longus ____
    c) tibialis anterior ____
    d) tibialis posterior ____
    e) popliteus ____

The Musculoskeletal System

53. a) **FALSE** The intertrochanteric line lies anteriorly; the intertrochanteric crest lies posteriorly.
    b) **FALSE** Posteriorly, the capsule is attached halfway along the neck.
    c) **TRUE** The muscle winds round the inferior aspect to reach the trochanteric fossa.
    d) **TRUE** The blood supply to the head of the femur reaches it through the neck.
    e) **FALSE** Marked lateral rotation of the thigh is a sign of a fractured neck of the femur.

54. a) **TRUE** The patella forms within the tendon of quadriceps femoris.
    b) **TRUE** And also by vastus medialis.
    c) **TRUE** These fibres are horizontal and help to stabilise the patella.
    d) **FALSE** The lateral facet of the patella is larger than the medial facet.
    e) **FALSE** The articular surface is lined by hyaline cartilage.

55. a) **FALSE** The popliteal artery is deeper and closer to the bone.
    b) **FALSE** The nerve is more superficial in the popliteal fossa.
    c) **TRUE**
    d) **FALSE** It winds round the neck of the fibula.
    e) **TRUE** It lies deep to quadraceps and covers the front of the lower end.

56. a) **TRUE** The extensor tendons become incorporated into the extensor expansion on the dorsal surface of each toe.
    b) **FALSE** Flexor digitorum longus arises from the tibia below the soleal line.
    c) **FALSE** Tibialis anterior originates from the lateral surface of the tibia.
    d) **TRUE** The tendon of tibialis posterior passes behind the medial malleolus.
    e) **FALSE** Popliteus attaches to the tibia above the soleal line.

The Musculoskeletal System

57. The talus articulates with
 a) the navicular
 b) the calcaneus
 c) the cuboid
 d) the medial cuneiform
 e) the lateral cuneiform

58. The following structures are attached to the talus:
 a) the deltoid ligament
 b) the long plantar ligament
 c) tibialis posterior
 d) extensor pollicis brevis
 e) the spring ligament

59. With regard to the quadriceps femoris muscle:
 a) the rectus femoris component functions as a flexor at the hip
 b) the main functional attachment at the lower end is into the tibia via the ligamentum patellae
 c) its nerve supply comes from the lumbar spinal nerves
 d) the lowermost fibres of the vastus medialis muscle are almost horizontally arranged
 e) the lower part is related to the suprapatellar bursa

60. The hamstring muscles
 a) are all innervated by the peroneal component of the sciatic nerve
 b) extend the thigh at the hip joint
 c) extend the thigh on the knee joint if the leg is fixed
 d) limit extension at the knee joint if the thigh is flexed
 e) limit flexion of the hip when the knee is extended

57. a) **TRUE** The head of the talus articulates anteriorly with the navicular.
    b) **TRUE** The sinus tarsi between the talus and calcaneum transmits the interosseous talocalcaneal ligament.
    c) **FALSE**
    d) **FALSE**
    e) **FALSE** The cuneiform bones articulate proximally with the navicular bone.

58. a) **TRUE** It is attached to the side of the talus.
    b) **FALSE** It is attached to the calcaneum, the cuboid and the metatarsal bones.
    c) **FALSE** It is attached to all the tarsal bones except the talus.
    d) **FALSE** The talus has no muscle attachment and hence has a poor blood supply.
    e) **FALSE** The spring ligament supports the head of the talus, but is not attached to it.

59. a) **TRUE** It is attached to the hip bone.
    b) **TRUE** It is attached to the tibial tuberosity.
    c) **TRUE** Through the femoral nerve.
    d) **TRUE** They are attached to the patella and help to stabilise the patella.
    e) **TRUE** This bursa separates the muscle from the femur.

60. a) **FALSE** All are innervated by the tibial nerve except the short head of biceps which is innervated by the common peroneal nerve.
    b) **TRUE** Gluteus maximus is another extensor.
    c) **FALSE** They are flexors of the knee.
    d) **TRUE** In this position the hamstrings are stretched.
    e) **TRUE** Again, the hamstrings are stretched in this position.

The Musculoskeletal System

61. A CT scan midway between the hip and knee joints shows
   a) rectus femoris anterior to vastus medialis and intermedius
   b) the fleshy belly of semimembranosus
   c) the psoas tendon
   d) the sartorius and the femoral vessels
   e) the femoral nerve

62. The following are attached to the tendocalcaneus:
   a) soleus muscle
   b) gastrocnemius muscle
   c) flexor hallucis longus muscle
   d) tibialis posterior tendon
   e) plantaris

63. The tibialis posterior muscle
   a) has a tendon with no synovial sheath
   b) is an invertor of the foot
   c) has a tendon which grooves the back of the lateral malleolus
   d) is inserted chiefly distal to the subtalar joint
   e) is supplied by the deep peroneal nerve

64. With regard to muscles in the posterior compartment of the leg:
   a) they include flexors at the knee joint
   b) all are innervated by the tibial nerve
   c) they include invertors of the foot
   d) they are inactive in maintenance of the resting erect posture
   e) only tibialis posterior has an attachment to the tibia

The Musculoskeletal System

61. a) **TRUE**
 b) **TRUE**
 c) **FALSE** The psoas tendon is inserted into the lesser trochanter.
 d) **TRUE**
 e) **FALSE** The femoral nerve divides into its branches higher up in the thigh.

62. a) **TRUE**
 b) **TRUE**
 c) **FALSE**
 d) **FALSE**
 e) **TRUE**

63. a) **FALSE** All tendons in the foot have synovial sheaths.
 b) **TRUE** Tibialis anterior and posterior are the main invertors.
 c) **FALSE** The tendon lies behind the medial malleolus.
 d) **TRUE** Its main insertion is into the tuberosity of the navicular bone.
 e) **FALSE** All the muscles in the posterior compartment of the leg are innervated by the tibial nerve.

64. a) **TRUE** Gastrocnemius can flex the knee.
 b) **TRUE**
 c) **TRUE**
 d) **FALSE** Their activity, especially that of soleus, is essential for maintaining erect posture.
 e) **FALSE** Flexor digitorum longus and soleus also have attachments to the tibia.

The Musculoskeletal System

65. **The pull of the superficial muscles of the calf may avulse a portion of the bone(s) into which they are inserted, namely**
    a) the tibia
    b) the fibula
    c) the talus
    d) the calcaneus
    e) the cuneiform

66. **The soleus muscle**
    a) lies deep to the gastrocnemius muscle
    b) arises from the tibia only
    c) is supplied by the common peroneal nerve
    d) contains few veins
    e) has a common insertion with the flexor hallucis longus

67. **The sacro-iliac joint**
    a) is a fibrocartilaginous joint
    b) transmits the body weight to the lower limb
    c) ligaments are important in stabilising the joint
    d) ligaments are important in weight bearing
    e) sacrotuberous ligament is attached to the ischial spine

68. **The hip joint owes its stability to**
    a) the diameter of the femoral head being greater than the rim of the acetabular labrum
    b) a thick and tight fibrous capsule
    c) the tautness of the iliofemoral ligament in extension
    d) the strength of the ligament of the head of the femur
    e) the short lateral rotators of the femur

The Musculoskeletal System

65. a) **FALSE**
b) **FALSE**
c) **FALSE**
d) **TRUE**
e) **FALSE**

66. a) **TRUE**
b) **FALSE** Soleus also arises from the fibula.
c) **FALSE** It is supplied by the tibial nerve.
d) **TRUE** Contraction of soleus is important in venous return from the leg.
e) **FALSE** Soleus forms the tendocalcaneus with gastrocnemius and plantaris.

67. a) **FALSE** The sacro-iliac joint is a synovial joint.
b) **TRUE**
c) **TRUE**
d) **TRUE**
e) **FALSE** The sacrotuberous ligament is attached to the ischial tuberosity.

68. a) **TRUE** The bony surfaces make a good fit as the smaller size of the rim prevents the head from slipping out of the acetabulum.
b) **TRUE** The capsule is thicker and tighter than that of the shoulder joint.
c) **TRUE** This is the strongest ligament in the body.
d) **TRUE**
e) **TRUE** These muscles are closely related to the capsule.

The Musculoskeletal System

69. **In radiographs of the hip joint in the anatomical position**
    a) the tip of the greater trochanter is in the same horizontal plane as the middle of the femur
    b) the tip of the greater trochanter is in the same horizontal plane as the pubic tubercle
    c) the inferior surfaces of the femoral neck and head form a curve continuous with the superior ramus of the pubis (Shenton's line)
    d) the ischial tuberosity is in the same horizontal plane as the tip of the greater trochanter
    e) the lesser trochanter is not visible

70. **The knee joint**
    a) is essentially a modified hinge joint with an ability to rotate when extended
    b) is reinforced medially by the tibial collateral ligament
    c) contains cruciate ligaments which lie within the synovial cavity
    d) receives its nerve supply from the femoral and sciatic nerves
    e) has a lateral meniscus to which popliteus is attached posteriorly

71. **The capsule of the knee joint**
    a) is reinforced by expansions from surrounding muscles and tendons
    b) is penetrated by the cruciate ligaments
    c) is attached to both the menisci at their peripheral margins
    d) is pierced by the tendon of popliteus
    e) is pierced by the genicular nerves and vessels

The Musculoskeletal System

69. a) **FALSE** It lies in the same plane as the head of the femur.
   b) **FALSE** It is in the same horizontal plane as the upper border of the pubic symphysis.
   c) **TRUE** This is altered when the joint is dislocated.
   d) **FALSE** The tip of the greater trochanter lies in the same plane as the spine of the ischium.
   e) **FALSE** Both trochanters are visible.

70. a) **TRUE**
   b) **TRUE**
   c) **FALSE** They are intracapsular but extrasynovial.
   d) **TRUE** And also from the obturator nerve.
   e) **TRUE** This makes the meniscus more mobile.

71. a) **TRUE**
   b) **FALSE** The cruciate ligaments are intracapsular.
   c) **FALSE** It is attached only to the medial meniscus.
   d) **TRUE** The muscle takes origin from inside the joint.
   e) **TRUE**

The Musculoskeletal System

72. Blood from the knee joint can be aspirated through
   a) the prepatellar bursa
   b) the deep infrapatellar bursa
   c) the suprapatellar bursa
   d) the superficial infrapatellar bursa
   e) the semimembranosus bursa

73. The anterior cruciate ligament
   a) is attached to the lateral surface of the medial condyle of the femur
   b) is taut in full extension
   c) prevents the tibia sliding forwards on the femur
   d) is attached to the anterior part of the intercondylar region of the tibia
   e) is intrasynovial

74. The medial (deltoid) ligament is attached to
   a) the medial malleolus
   b) the sustentaculum tali
   c) the spring ligament
   d) the tuberosity of the navicular
   e) the calcaneus

75. Inversion and eversion of the foot take place at
   a) the ankle joint
   b) the talofibular joint
   c) the talonavicular joint
   d) the subtalar joint
   e) the metatarsophalangeal joint

76. The longitudinal arch of the foot is supported by
   a) the plantar aponeurosis
   b) the spring ligament
   c) the sustentaculum tali
   d) the tendocalcaneus
   e) the flexor hallucis longus

The Musculoskeletal System

72. a) **FALSE**
    b) **FALSE**
    c) **TRUE**
    d) **FALSE**
    e) **FALSE**

73. a) **FALSE** It is attached to the medial surface of the lateral condyle.
    b) **TRUE**
    c) **TRUE**
    d) **TRUE**
    e) **FALSE**

74. a) **TRUE**
    b) **TRUE**
    c) **TRUE**
    d) **TRUE**
    e) **TRUE** It is attached to the sustentaculum tali.

75. a) **FALSE**
    b) **FALSE**
    c) **TRUE**
    d) **TRUE**
    e) **FALSE**

76. a) **TRUE**
    b) **TRUE**
    c) **FALSE**
    d) **FALSE**
    e) **TRUE**

The Musculoskeletal System

77. **With regard to the leg and foot:**
    a) compound fractures of the tibia are rare
    b) the talus has a relatively poor blood supply
    c) peroneus brevis everts the foot
    d) the plantar calcaneonavicular ('spring') ligament articulates by a synovial joint with the cuneiform
    e) the calcaneofibular ligament may be torn if the foot is forcefully inverted

The Musculoskeletal System

77. a) **FALSE**   Such fractures are very common, as the anteromedial surface of the tibia is subcutaneous.
    b) **TRUE**   It has no muscle attachments and most surfaces are covered by articular cartilage.
    c) **TRUE**   Both the peronei are evertors of the foot.
    d) **FALSE**   It articulates with the head of the talus.
    e) **TRUE**

The Musculoskeletal System

THE HEAD AND NECK

True/False

78. With regard to the sutures of the skull:
  a) they are fibrous joints between skull bones
  b) they are present throughout life
  c) the coronal suture separates the frontal bone from the temporal bones
  d) the sagittal suture separates the two parietal bones
  e) the lambdoid suture separates the occipital bone from the parietal bones

79. The anterior fontanelle is
  a) open for 2 years
  b) larger than the posterior fontanelle
  c) above the superior sagittal sinus
  d) a site through which cerebrospinal fluid can be withdrawn
  e) depressed when the patient is dehydrated

80. The pituitary (hypophyseal) fossa
  a) forms part of the middle cranial fossa
  b) lies above the body of the sphenoid
  c) is readily visible in lateral radiographs of the skull
  d) is lined by dura, arachnoid and pia mater
  e) is closely related to the cavernous sinus

81. With regard to the pituitary (hypophyseal) fossa:
  a) dura (diaphragma sellae) forms the roof
  b) the sphenoidal sinus lies between the nasal cavity and the hypophyseal fossa
  c) it contains the pituitary and the pineal glands
  d) it is bounded in part by the anterior clinoid processes
  e) the cavernous sinus lies in front of the fossa

The Musculoskeletal System

THE HEAD AND NECK

78. a) **TRUE**
    b) **FALSE** They are converted to bone in old age.
    c) **FALSE** It separates the frontal bone from the parietal bones.
    d) **TRUE**
    e) **TRUE**

79. a) **FALSE** The anterior fontanelle closes by about 18 months, after the posterior fontanelle which closes at the end of the first year.
    b) **TRUE** The anterior is the larger of the fontanelles.
    c) **TRUE** Blood can be withdrawn through the fontanelle.
    d) **TRUE** This can be done by putting the needle lateral to the sinus.
    e) **TRUE** And it bulges out when the intracranial tension is increased.

80. a) **TRUE** It lies in the middle part of the middle cranial fossa.
    b) **TRUE**
    c) **TRUE** It lies above the sphenoidal sinus.
    d) **FALSE** The hypophyseal fossa is lined only by the dura mater.
    e) **TRUE**

81. a) **TRUE**
    b) **TRUE**
    c) **FALSE** It contains only the pituitary gland.
    d) **TRUE** It is also bounded by the posterior clinoid processes.
    e) **FALSE** The cavernous sinuses lie on either side of the fossa.

The Musculoskeletal System

82. The foramen ovale transmits
   a) the maxillary artery _____
   b) the greater petrosal nerve _____
   c) emissary veins _____
   d) the accessory middle meningeal artery _____
   e) the mandibular nerve _____

83. Fractures of the sphenoid bone may include
   a) the anterior clinoid process _____
   b) the internal auditory meatus _____
   c) the medial pterygoid plate _____
   d) the optic canal _____
   e) the foramen spinosum _____

84. The optic canal transmits
   a) the optic nerve _____
   b) the ophthalmic veins _____
   c) the oculomotor nerve _____
   d) the ophthalmic artery _____
   e) the infraorbital nerve _____

85. The superior orbital fissure transmits
   a) the abducens nerve _____
   b) the trochlear nerve _____
   c) the lacrimal nerve _____
   d) the maxillary nerve _____
   e) the ciliary nerves _____

86. The middle cranial fossa is formed by the following bones:
   a) petrous temporal _____
   b) squamous temporal _____
   c) cribriform plate of the ethmoid _____
   d) basilar part of the occipital _____
   e) greater wing of the sphenoid _____

The Musculoskeletal System

82. a) **FALSE**
    b) **FALSE**
    c) **TRUE**
    d) **TRUE**
    e) **TRUE**

83. a) **TRUE** It is part of the lesser wing of sphenoid.
    b) **FALSE** It is on the temporal bone.
    c) **TRUE**
    d) **TRUE**
    e) **TRUE** It is on the greater wing of the sphenoid.

84. a) **TRUE** And also all three layers of the meninges surrounding the nerve.
    b) **FALSE** The ophthalmic veins go through the superior orbital fissure to drain into the cavernous sinus.
    c) **FALSE** The two divisions of the oculomotor nerve go through the superior orbital fissure.
    d) **TRUE** It lies on the inferolateral aspect of the optic nerve.
    e) **FALSE** It passes through the infraorbital canal.

85. a) **TRUE** It supplies the lateral rectus.
    b) **TRUE** It supplies the superior oblique.
    c) **TRUE** It is a branch of the ophthalmic division of the trigeminal nerve.
    d) **FALSE** It goes through the foramen rotundum.
    e) **FALSE** These are branches of the nasociliary nerve in the orbit.

86. a) **TRUE**
    b) **TRUE**
    c) **FALSE** It is in the anterior cranial fossa.
    d) **FALSE** It is in the posterior cranial fossa.
    e) **TRUE**

The Musculoskeletal System

87. The temporal bone
   a) is entirely in the middle cranial fossa
   b) contains the internal auditory meatus
   c) transmits the facial nerve
   d) has the falx cerebri attached to it
   e) has the tentorium cerebelli attached to it

88. The occipital bone
   a) possesses a groove for the transverse sinus
   b) has a pharyngeal tubercle
   c) contains the internal auditory meatus
   d) contains the anterior condylar canal
   e) contains the carotid canal

89. The posterior cranial fossa
   a) has a floor in a plane below that of the middle cranial fossa
   b) contains the abducens nerve
   c) contains the basilar artery
   d) contains part of the internal carotid artery
   e) contains the posterior clinoid processes

90. The internal acoustic meatus transmits
   a) the posterior inferior cerebellar artery
   b) the facial nerve
   c) the vestibulocochlear nerve
   d) the nervus intermedius
   e) the labyrinthine artery

91. The jugular foramen contains
   a) the superior petrosal sinus
   b) the glossopharyngeal nerve
   c) the vagus nerve
   d) the hypoglossal nerve
   e) the accessory nerve

The Musculoskeletal System

87. a) **FALSE** The posterior surface of the petrous part of the temporal bone is in the posterior cranial fossa.
    b) **TRUE** It is on the petrous temporal bone.
    c) **TRUE** The vestibulocochlear nerve accompanies it.
    d) **FALSE**
    e) **TRUE** The tentorium is attached to the petrous temporal bone.

88. a) **TRUE** And also for the sigmoid sinus.
    b) **TRUE**
    c) **FALSE**
    d) **TRUE** This transmits the hypoglossal nerve.
    e) **FALSE** It is in the petrous part of the temporal bone.

89. a) **TRUE**
    b) **TRUE** All the lower cranial nerves traverse the fossa.
    c) **TRUE** It lies on the pons, which is in the fossa.
    d) **FALSE** It is in the middle cranial fossa.
    e) **TRUE** These lie at the border between the middle and the posterior fossae.

90. a) **FALSE**
    b) **TRUE**
    c) **TRUE**
    d) **TRUE**
    e) **TRUE**

91. a) **FALSE** The superior petrosal sinus joins the transverse sinus. The jugular foramen transmits the inferior petrosal sinus.
    b) **TRUE**
    c) **TRUE**
    d) **FALSE**
    e) **TRUE**

The Musculoskeletal System

92. **The styloid process**
    a) is a fibrocartilaginous structure
    b) is derived from the third pharyngeal arch
    c) is closely related to the facial nerve
    d) is connected to the hyoid bone by a muscle and a ligament
    e) lies between the parotid gland and the carotid sheath

93. **The mastoid process**
    a) is fully developed at birth
    b) contains air cells in communication with the middle ear cavity
    c) has the sternohyoid and sternomastoid muscles attached to the external surface
    d) is closely related to the facial nerve
    e) lies anterior to the external auditory meatus

94. **Air cells are usually found in**
    a) the frontal bone
    b) the temporal bone
    c) the maxilla
    d) the parietal bone
    e) the occipital bone

95. **The stylomastoid foramen**
    a) lies medial to the styloid process
    b) transmits the facial nerve
    c) transmits the chorda tympani
    d) transmits the middle meningeal vessels
    e) is very superficial in the newborn

The Musculoskeletal System

92. a) **FALSE** It is part of the temporal bone.
    b) **FALSE** It is a derivative of the second arch.
    c) **TRUE** The stylomastoid foramen transmitting the nerve lies posterior to the styloid process.
    d) **TRUE** By the stylohyoid muscle and stylohyoid ligament.
    e) **TRUE** The styloid process and associated structures separate the two.

93. a) **FALSE** It develops fully after birth.
    b) **TRUE** Through the mastoid antrum.
    c) **FALSE** The sternohyoid is attached to the hyoid bone.
    d) **TRUE** The stylomastoid foramen transmits the nerve.
    e) **FALSE** The mastoid process lies posterior to the meatus.

94. a) **TRUE** In the frontal sinuses.
    b) **TRUE** The mastoid air cells.
    c) **FALSE** The maxillary sinus is bigger than air cells.
    d) **FALSE**
    e) **FALSE**

95. a) **FALSE** It is lateral and slightly posterior to the styloid process.
    b) **TRUE**
    c) **FALSE** The chorda tympani comes out through the petrotympanic fissure.
    d) **FALSE** These vessels are transmitted through the foramen spinosum.
    e) **TRUE** Because the mastoid is not developed.

The Musculoskeletal System

96. With regard to the mandible:
   a) the lateral pterygoid is attached to the ramus _____
   b) masseter is attached to the ramus _____
   c) it has the groove for the nerve to mylohyoid on its medial surface _____
   d) the submandibular gland lies entirely below the mylohyoid line _____
   e) the mental foramen may be palpated under the tongue _____

97. The mandible is closely related to
   a) the hypoglossal nerve _____
   b) the lingual nerve _____
   c) the auriculotemporal nerve _____
   d) the inferior alveolar nerve _____
   e) the vagus nerve _____

98. Concerning the temporomandibular joint:
   a) it is supplied by the maxillary nerve _____
   b) fibrocartilage covers the articular surface _____
   c) its capsule is attached behind the squamotympanic fissure _____
   d) the mouth is opened by the medial pterygoid muscle _____
   e) side-to-side movement is produced by the medial pterygoid muscle _____

99. The medial pterygoid muscle
   a) is innervated by the mandibular nerve _____
   b) is easily palpable _____
   c) has an attachment to the temporomandibular joint articular disc _____
   d) takes origin from the medial pterygoid plate _____
   e) is closely related to the lingual nerve _____

The Musculoskeletal System

96. a) **FALSE** It is the medial pterygoid which is attached to the medial surface of the ramus.
    b) **TRUE** To its outer aspect.
    c) **TRUE**
    d) **FALSE** The deep part of the gland lies above the mylohyoid muscle and hence above the line.
    e) **FALSE** The mental foramen is on the lateral surface of the mandible.

97. a) **FALSE** The hypoglossal nerve lies on the hyoglossus but not close to the mandible.
    b) **TRUE** The lingual nerve lies very close to the medial aspect of the last molar tooth.
    c) **TRUE** This nerve passes close to the neck of the mandible.
    d) **TRUE** It goes through the mandibular canal.
    e) **FALSE** The vagus lies in the carotid sheath.

98. a) **FALSE** It is supplied by the auriculotemporal nerve and the nerve to masseter.
    b) **TRUE** Unlike many other synovial joints.
    c) **FALSE** It is attached to the anterior lip of the fissure.
    d) **FALSE** It is opened by the lateral pterygoid muscle.
    e) **TRUE**

99. a) **TRUE** All the muscles of mastication are innervated by the mandibular nerve.
    b) **FALSE** As it is medial to the ramus of the mandible.
    c) **FALSE** It is the lateral pterygoid that has an attachment to the temporomandibular joint articular disc.
    d) **FALSE** It takes origin from the medial surface of the lateral pterygoid plate.
    e) **TRUE** The lingual and inferior alveolar nerves lie on its external surface.

The Musculoskeletal System

100. **The function of the medial pterygoid muscle is to assist other muscles in**
    a) elevating the jaw
    b) retracting the jaw
    c) protruding the jaw
    d) moving the jaw laterally to the ipsilateral side
    e) moving the jaw laterally to the contralateral side

101. **Muscles that close the jaw include**
    a) temporalis
    b) buccinator
    c) medial pterygoid
    d) lateral pterygoid
    e) mylohyoid

102. **The lateral pterygoid muscle**
    a) is attached to the medial pterygoid plate
    b) is attached to the condyle of the mandible
    c) is attached to the capsule of the temporomandibular joint
    d) is supplied by the anterior division of the mandibular nerve
    e) contracts to cause retraction of the mandible

103. **The lateral pterygoid**
    a) has a venous plexus on it
    b) is derived from the second branchial arch
    c) arises from the lateral side of the lateral pterygoid plate
    d) is crossed by the maxillary artery
    e) has the mandibular nerve deep to it

The Musculoskeletal System

100. a) **TRUE** It acts along with masseter and temporalis.
b) **FALSE** Retraction of the jaw is mostly by the posterior fibres of temporalis.
c) **FALSE** The lateral pterygoid is mainly responsible for jaw protrusion.
d) **FALSE**
e) **TRUE**

101. a) **TRUE**
b) **FALSE**
c) **TRUE**
d) **FALSE** The lateral pterygoid is involved in opening the mouth.
e) **FALSE** This muscle may also be involved in opening the mouth.

102. a) **FALSE** It is attached to the lateral surface of the lateral pterygoid plate.
b) **TRUE** It is attached to the pterygoid fovea on the upper part of the neck.
c) **TRUE** And also to the articular disc.
d) **TRUE** Most of the muscles of mastication are supplied by the anterior division.
e) **FALSE**

103. a) **TRUE** The pterygoid muscles are closely related to the pterygoid plexus of veins.
b) **FALSE** The muscles of mastication are derived from the first arch.
c) **TRUE**
d) **TRUE** The artery may cross it on its lateral or medial surface.
e) **TRUE** The trunk of the nerve is deep to the muscle.

The Musculoskeletal System

104. The mylohyoid muscle
   a) is attached to the inferior border of the mandible
   b) is pierced by the submandibular duct
   c) is pierced by the lingual nerve
   d) is supplied by the hypoglossal nerve
   e) contracts to raise the floor of the mouth

105. The mylohyoid muscle
   a) is related to the anterior belly of digastric
   b) is attached to the thyroid cartilage
   c) plays a part in mastication
   d) has the submandibular gland lying between it and the mandible
   e) has the sublingual gland lying deep to it

106. The sternocleidomastoid muscle
   a) is supplied by the accessory nerve and the second and third cervical nerves
   b) flexes the neck and rotates the face to the opposite side
   c) has two heads of origin
   d) lies medial to the phrenic nerve
   e) is crossed on its deep surface by the external jugular vein

107. With regard to scalenus anterior:
   a) it arises from the bodies of all the cervical vertebrae
   b) the subclavian vein is posterior to it
   c) the prevertebral fascia is anterior to it
   d) the phrenic nerve lies anterior to it
   e) the roots of the brachial plexus are anterior to it

The Musculoskeletal System

104. a) **FALSE** It is attached to the mylohyoid line on the inner surface of the mandible.
  b) **FALSE** The duct starts deep to the muscle from the deep part of the submandibular gland.
  c) **FALSE** The nerve lies deep to the mylohyoid on the hyoglossus.
  d) **FALSE** It is supplied by the mandibular nerve.
  e) **TRUE** This happens in swallowing.

105. a) **TRUE** The anterior belly of digastric lies on the inferior surface of the mylohyoid.
  b) **FALSE** It is attached to the hyoid bone.
  c) **TRUE** It helps to open the mouth.
  d) **TRUE** The deep part of the gland also lies deep to the muscle.
  e) **TRUE**

106. a) **TRUE** The motor supply is by the spinal accessory nerve; the sensory supply is by the second and third cervical nerves.
  b) **TRUE** It acts on the atlanto-axial joint.
  c) **TRUE** Sternal and clavicular heads.
  d) **FALSE** The phrenic nerve lying on scalenus anterior is deep to sternocleidomastoid.
  e) **FALSE** The external jugular vein is superficial.

107. a) **FALSE** It arises from the third to the sixth cervical vertebrae.
  b) **FALSE** The vein lies anterior and the artery posterior to the muscle.
  c) **TRUE** The scalene muscles are lined by the prevertebral fascia.
  d) **TRUE** It crosses it from lateral to medial.
  e) **FALSE** They are posterior, lying between scalenus anterior and scalenus medius.

The Musculoskeletal System

108. Concerning the suprahyoid muscles:
   a) geniohyoid is attached to the inferior genial tubercle ____
   b) they open the mouth against resistance ____
   c) they are supplied by the ansa cervicalis ____
   d) they raise the hyoid in swallowing ____
   e) geniohyoid is superficial to mylohyoid ____

109. Concerning the infrahyoid muscles:
   a) omohyoid is one of them ____
   b) they raise the thyroid gland in swallowing ____
   c) they separate the thyroid gland from the trachea ____
   d) they stabilise the hyoid to open the mouth against resistance ____
   e) they are supplied by the ansa cervicalis ____

The Musculoskeletal System

108. a) **TRUE**
  b) **TRUE**
  c) **FALSE** Geniohyoid is supplied by C1 through the hypoglossal nerve; the posterior belly of digastric and stylohyoid by the facial nerve; and mylohyoid and the anterior belly of digastric by the mandibular nerve.
  d) **TRUE**
  e) **FALSE** It lies deep to mylohyoid.

109. a) **TRUE**
  b) **FALSE** This is carried out by the suprahyoid muscles.
  c) **FALSE** They cover the gland superficially.
  d) **TRUE**
  e) **TRUE**

The Musculoskeletal System

Picture questions

Identify the numbered structures in the following illustrations from the choices given

Question 1(i)
1. ____
2. ____
3. ____
4. ____
5. ____
6. ____

    A. Foramen transversarium
    B. Transverse process
    C. Superior articular facet
    D. Anterior arch
    E. Synovial joint for dens
    F. Posterior arch

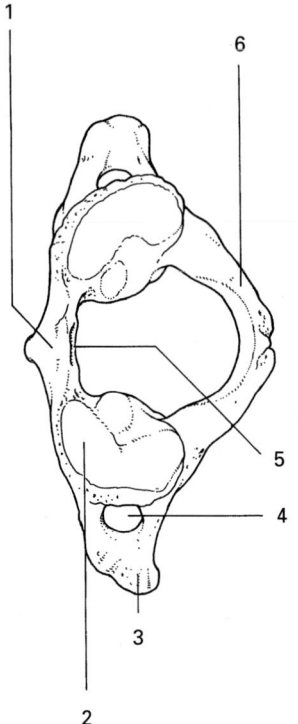

Question 1(ii)
1. ____
2. ____
3. ____
4. ____
5. ____

    A. Dens
    B. Spinous process
    C. Foramen transversarium
    D. Transverse process
    E. Superior articular facet

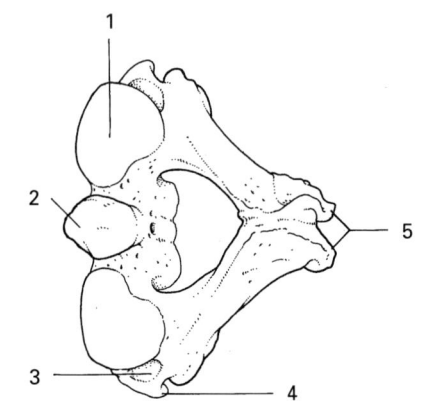

The Musculoskeletal System

Question 2
1. ____
2. ____
3. ____

A. Superior articular facet
B. Costovertebral joint
C. Costotransverse joint

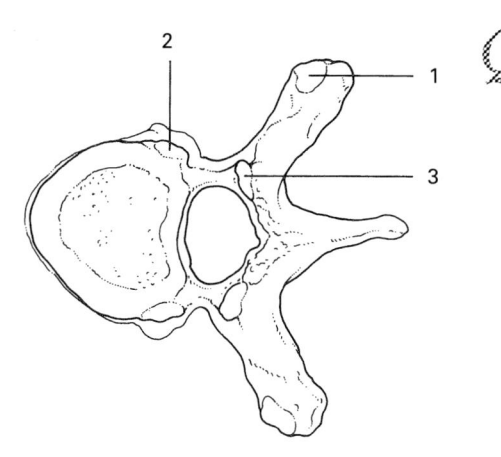

Question 3
1. ____
2. ____
3. ____
4. ____
5. ____

A. Costovertebral joint
B. Inferior articular facet
C. Costovertebral joint
D. Superior articular facet
E. Costotransverse joint

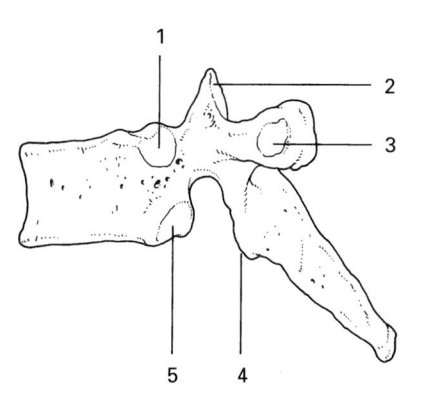

The Musculoskeletal System

Question 4
1. ____
2. ____
3. ____
4. ____
5. ____
6. ____
7. ____

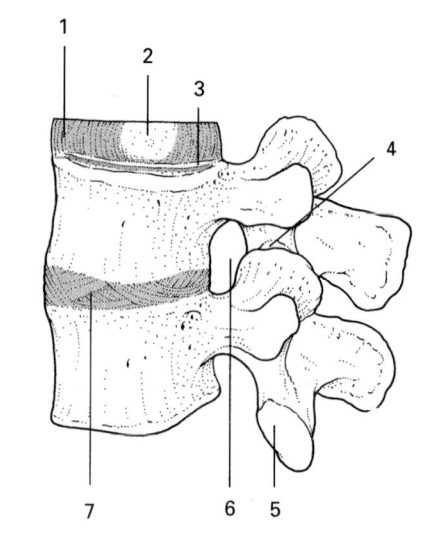

A. Nucleus pulposus
B. Intervertebral foramen
C. Annulus fibrosus
D. Hyaline cartilage
E. Inferior articular facet
F. Facet joint
G. Intervertebral disc

Question 5
1. ____
2. ____
3. ____
4. ____
5. ____
6. ____

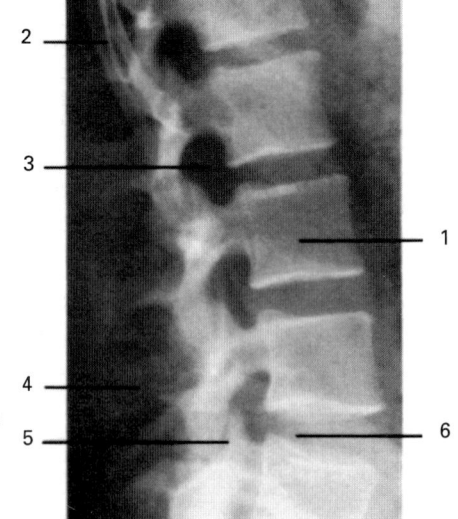

A. L4/L5 facet joint
B. Body of L3
C. Intervertebral foramen for second lumbar spinal nerve
D. L4/L5 disc space
E. Rib 12
F. L4 spinous process

The Musculoskeletal System

Question 6

1. ___
2. ___
3. ___
4. ___
5. ___
6. ___
7. ___
8. ___
9. ___
10. ___
11. ___
12. ___
13. ___
14. ___
15. ___
16. ___
17. ___
18. ___
19. ___
20. ___
21. ___
22. ___
23. ___

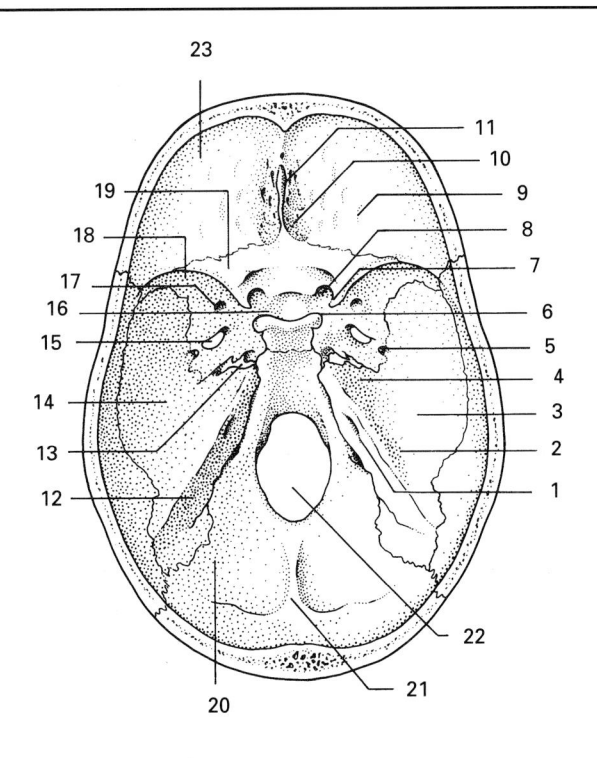

- **A.** Internal auditory meatus
- **B.** Squamous part of temporal bone
- **C.** Foramen spinosum
- **D.** Anterior clinoid process
- **E.** Optic canal
- **F.** Orbital plate of frontal bone
- **G.** Posterior clinoid process
- **H.** Tegmen tympani
- **I.** Arcuate eminence
- **J.** Middle cranial fossa
- **K.** Foramen lacerum
- **L.** Foramen magnum
- **M.** Internal occipital protruberance
- **N.** Cribriform plate
- **O.** Crista galli
- **P.** Greater wing of sphenoid
- **Q.** Hypophyseal fossa
- **R.** Foramen ovale
- **S.** Petrous part of temporal bone
- **T.** Posterior cranial fossa
- **U.** Lesser wing of sphenoid
- **V.** Anterior cranial fossa
- **W.** Foramen rotundum

Answers on pages 86 and 87

The Musculoskeletal System

Question 7

1. _____
2. _____
3. _____
4. _____
5. _____
6. _____
7. _____
8. _____
9. _____
10. _____
11. _____
12. _____
13. _____
14. _____
15. _____
16. _____
17. _____
18. _____
19. _____
20. _____

A. Inferior nuchal line
B. Alveolar process
C. Jugular foramen
D. Zygomatic arch
E. Horizontal plate of palatine bone
F. Palatal process of maxilla
G. Stylomastoid foramen
H. Pharyngeal tubercle
I. Groove for digastric muscle
J. Foramen spinosum
K. Foramen ovale
L. Lateral pterygoid plate
M. Greater palatine foramen
N. Occipital condyle
O. Foramen magnum
P. Mastoid process
Q. Incisor foramen
R. Carotid canal
S. Medial pterygoid plate
T. Styloid process

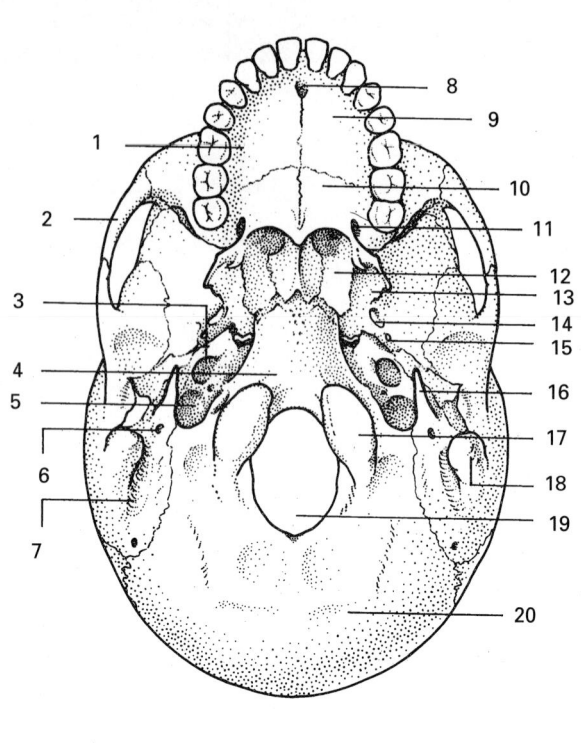

The Musculoskeletal System

Question 8
1. ____
2. ____
3. ____
4. ____
5. ____
6. ____
7. ____
8. ____
9. ____

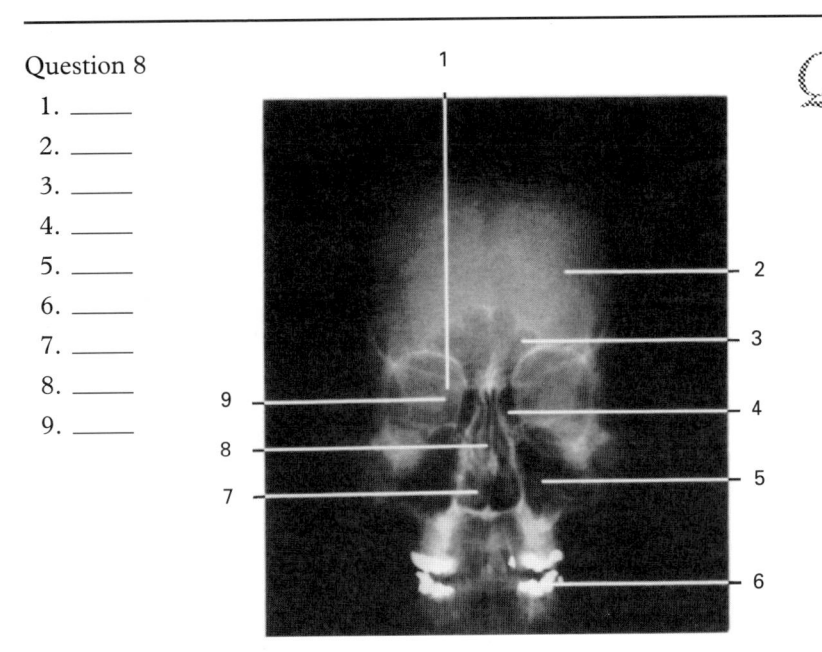

A. Lambdoid suture
B. Supraorbital fissure
C. Lesser wing of sphenoid
D. Fillings in teeth
E. Nasal septum
F. Frontal sinus
G. Maxillary sinus
H. Ethmoidal sinuses
I. Inferior concha

Answers on page 88

The Musculoskeletal System

Question 9
1. ____
2. ____
3. ____
4. ____
5. ____
6. ____
7. ____
8. ____
9. ____
10. ____
11. ____

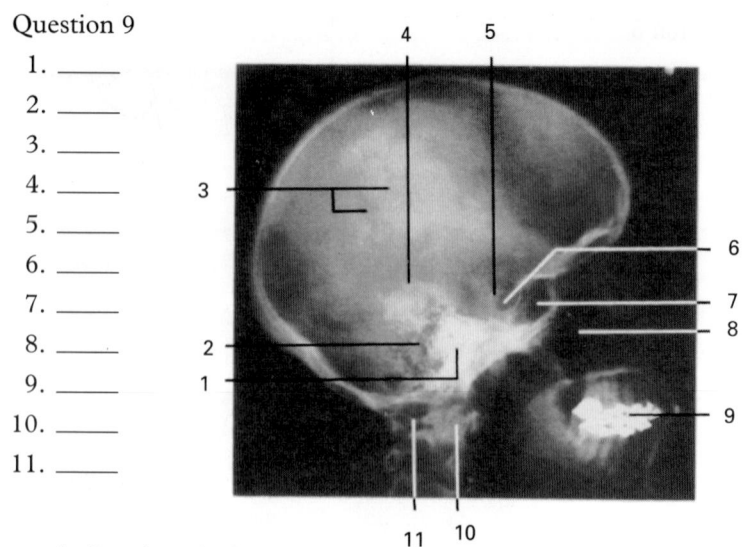

A. Posterior arch of atlas
B. Odontoid process of axis
C. Fillings in teeth
D. Petrous temporal bone
E. Grooves for middle meningeal vessels
F. Mastoid air cells
G. Maxillary sinus
H. Top of the ear
I. Posterior clinoid process
J. Sphenoid air sinus
K. Hypophyseal fossa

The Musculoskeletal System

Question 10

1. _____
2. _____
3. _____
4. _____
5. _____
6. _____
7. _____
8. _____
9. _____

A. Rectus capitis lateralis
B. Rectus capitis anterior
C. Apical pleura
D. Longus capitis
E. Scalenus anterior
F. Subclavian artery
G. Longus colli
H. Brachial plexus
I. Scalenus medius

Question 11

1. _____
2. _____
3. _____
4. _____
5. _____

A. Intercostal artery
B. Internal intercostals
C. Intercostal vein
D. External intercostals
E. Intercostal nerve

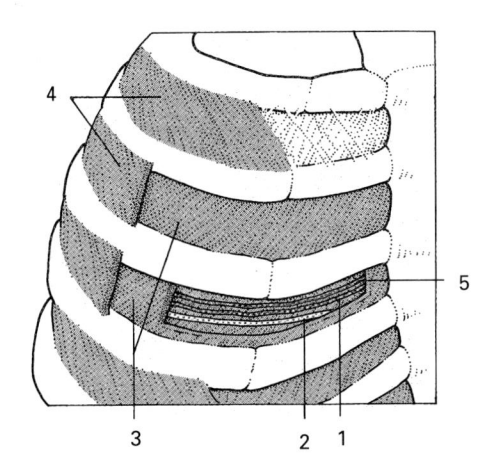

Answers on page 89

The Musculoskeletal System

Question 12

1. ____
2. ____
3. ____
4. ____
5. ____
6. ____
7. ____
8. ____
9. ____
10. ____
11. ____
12. ____
13. ____
14. ____
15. ____

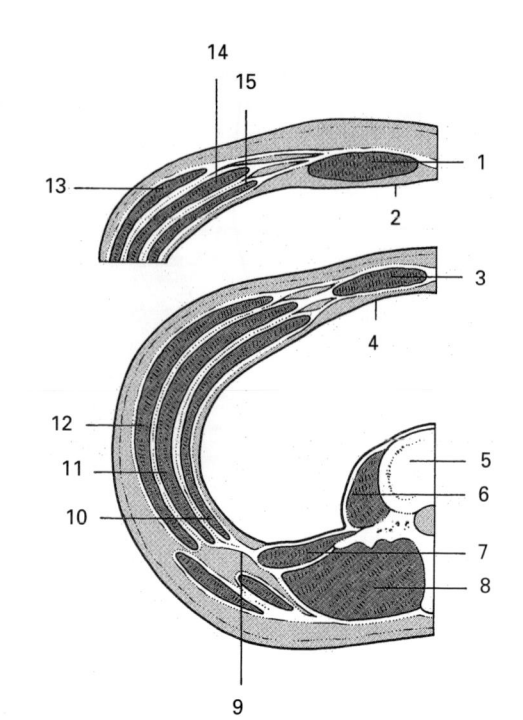

A. Lumbar vertebra
B. Transversalis fascia
C. Transversus abdominis
D. Internal oblique
E. External oblique
F. Quadratus lumborum
G. Psoas major
H. Rectus abdominis
I. Internal oblique
J. External oblique
K. Rectus abdominis
L. Transversus abdominis
M. Lumbar fascia
N. Erector spinae
O. Transversalis fascia

The Musculoskeletal System

Question 13
1. _____
2. _____
3. _____
4. _____

A. Inguinal ligament
B. External oblique
C. Rectus abdominis
D. Internal oblique

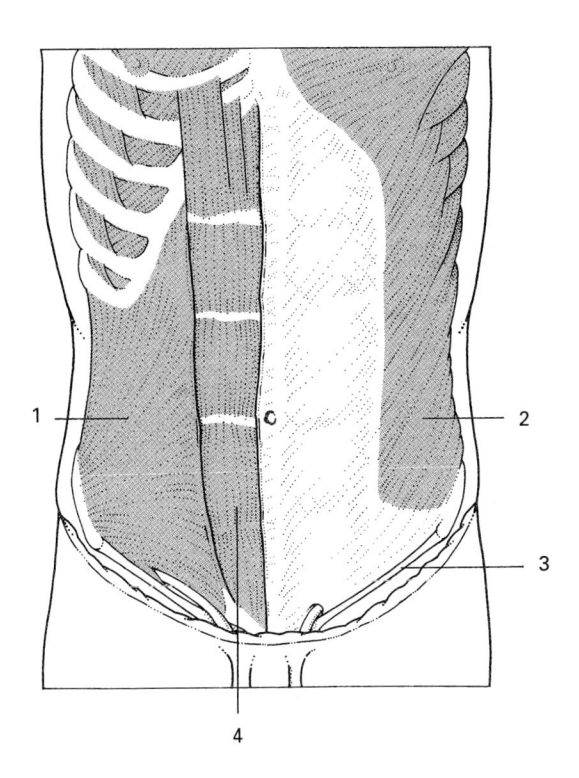

Answers on page 90

The Musculoskeletal System

Question 14

1. ____
2. ____
3. ____
4. ____
5. ____
6. ____
7. ____
8. ____
9. ____
10. ____
11. ____
12. ____
13. ____
14. ____
15. ____
16. ____
17. ____
18. ____
19. ____

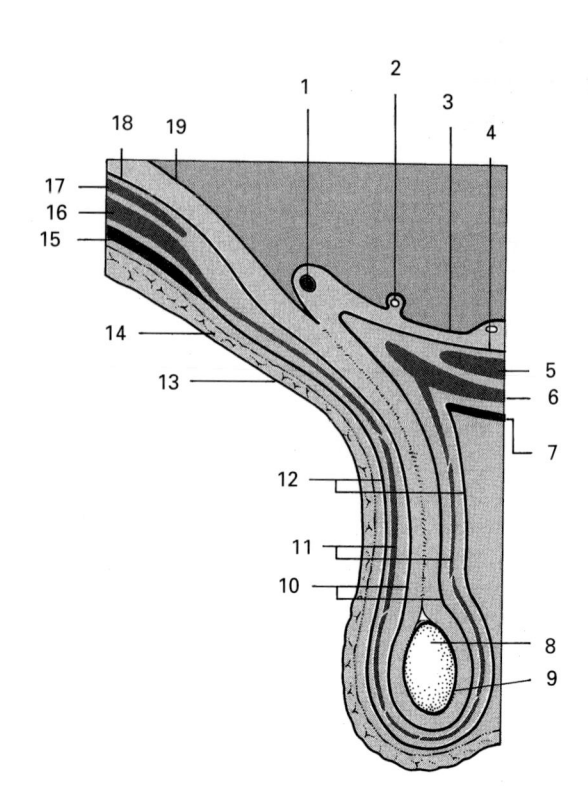

A. Obliterated umbilical artery
B. Transversalis fascia
C. Peritoneum
D. Inferior epigastric artery
E. Transversus abdominis
F. External spermatic fascia
G. Peritoneum
H. Rectus abdominis
I. Transversalis fascia
J. Internal oblique and transversus abdominis (fused together)
K. Internal oblique
L. Skin
M. Subcutaneous fat
N. External oblique
O. External oblique aponeurosis
P. Testis
Q. Tunica vaginalis (derived from peritoneum)
R. Cremaster
S. Internal spermatic fascia (from transversalis fascia)

72

The Musculoskeletal System

Question 15

1. ____
2. ____
3. ____
4. ____
5. ____
6. ____
7. ____
8. ____
9. ____
10. ____
11. ____
12. ____
13. ____
14. ____
15. ____
16. ____
17. ____
18. ____
19. ____
20. ____

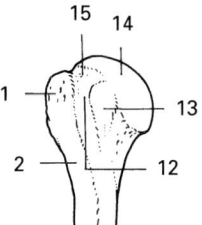

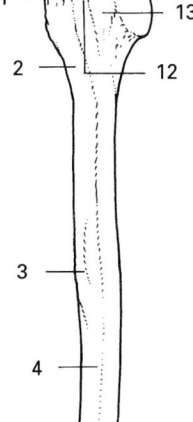

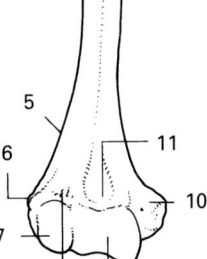

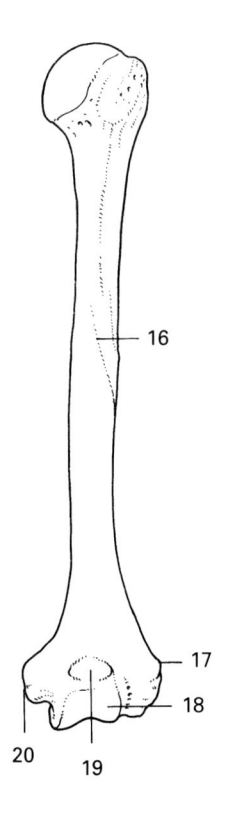

A. Capitulum
B. Radial fossa
C. Medial epicondyle
D. Coronoid fossa
E. Greater tuberosity (tubercle)
F. Surgical neck
G. Shaft
H. Deltoid tuberosity
I. Anatomical neck
J. Bicipital groove
K. Lateral supercondylar ridge
L. Head of humerus
M. Lesser tuberosity
N. Lateral epicondyle
O. Trochlea
P. Lateral epicondyle
Q. Spiral groove for radial nerve
R. Medial epicondyle
S. Olecranon fossa
T. Trochlea

Answers on pages 90 and 91   73

The Musculoskeletal System

Question 16

1. ____
2. ____
3. ____
4. ____
5. ____
6. ____
7. ____
8. ____
9. ____
10. ____
11. ____
12. ____

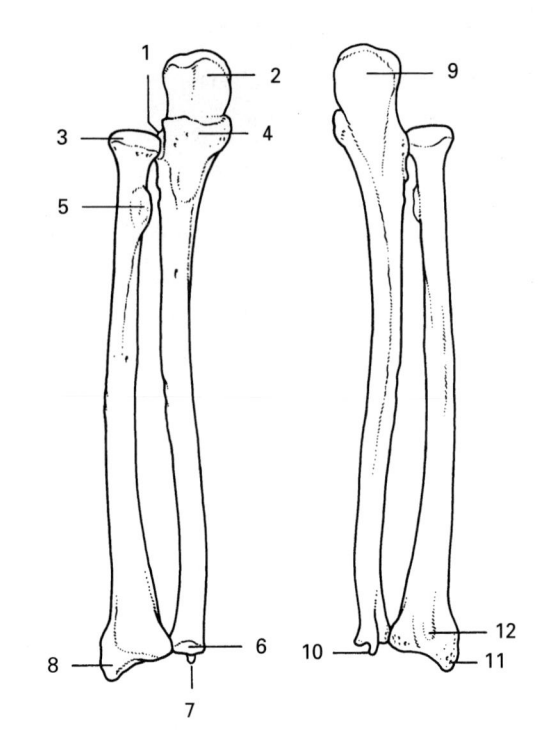

A. Styloid process of radius
B. Radial notch of ulna
C. Trochlear notch
D. Styloid process of radius
E. Head of radius
F. Head of ulna
G. Coronoid process
H. Styloid process of ulna
I. Dorsal tubercle
J. Olecranon
K. Radial tuberosity
L. Styloid process of ulna

The Musculoskeletal System

Question 17

1. _____
2. _____
3. _____
4. _____
5. _____
6. _____
7. _____
8. _____
9. _____
10. _____
11. _____
12. _____

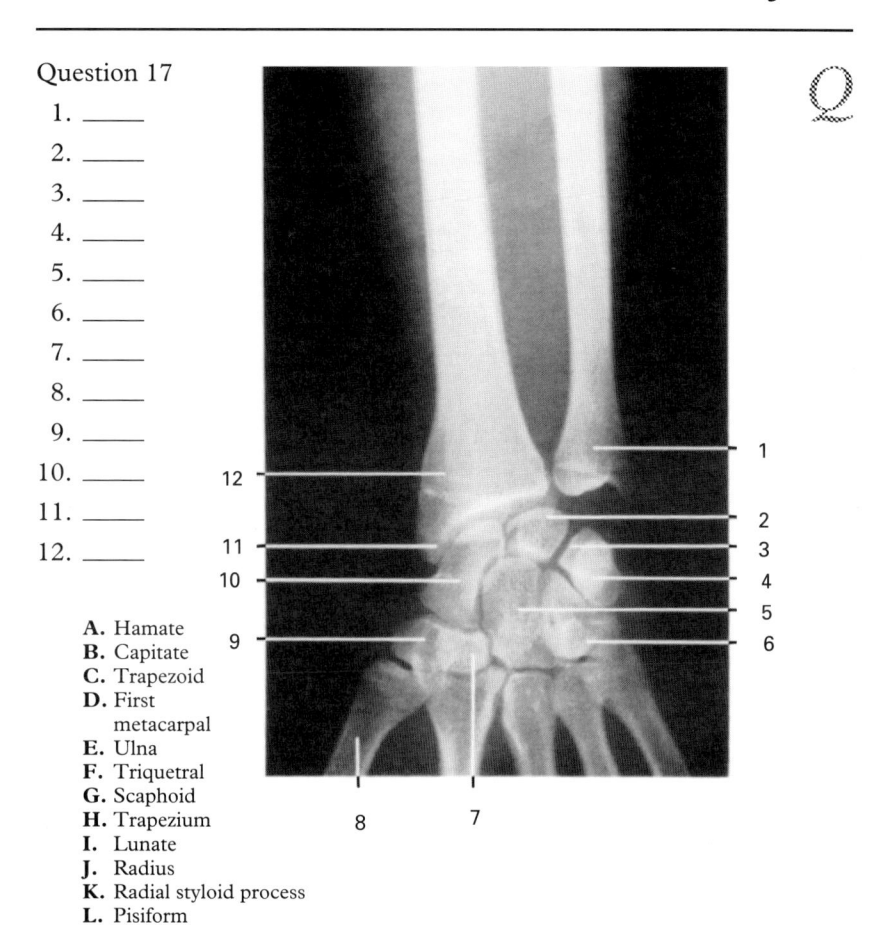

A. Hamate
B. Capitate
C. Trapezoid
D. First metacarpal
E. Ulna
F. Triquetral
G. Scaphoid
H. Trapezium
I. Lunate
J. Radius
K. Radial styloid process
L. Pisiform

Answers on pages 91 and 92

The Musculoskeletal System

Question 18

1. _____
2. _____
3. _____
4. _____
5. _____
6. _____

A. Supraspinatus
B. Infraspinatus
C. Teres minor
D. Deltoid
E. Teres major
F. Latissimus dorsi

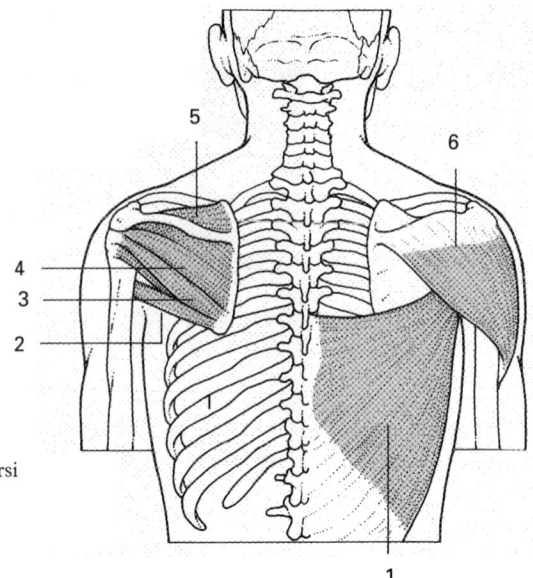

Question 19

1. _____
2. _____
3. _____
4. _____
5. _____

A. Flexor carpi ulnaris
B. Flexor carpi radialis
C. Palmaris longus
D. Pronator teres
E. Brachioradialis

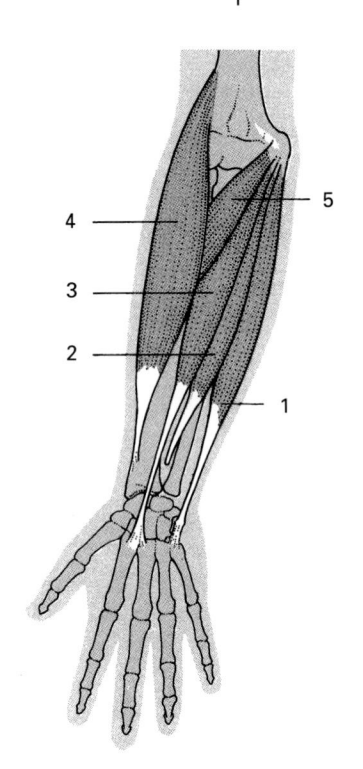

The Musculoskeletal System

Question 20
1. ____
2. ____
3. ____
4. ____

A. Fibrous flexor sheath
B. Flexor digitorum profundus
C. Flexor digitorum superficialis
D. Dorsal interosseus

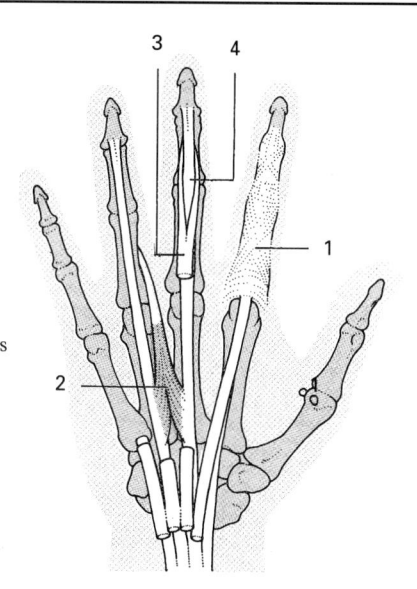

Question 21
1. ____
2. ____
3. ____
4. ____
5. ____

A. Fibrous flexor sheath
B. Flexor retinaculum
C. Synovial sheath for flexor tendons
D. Synovial sheath for flexor pollicis longus
E. Synovial sheath for flexor tendons to middle finger

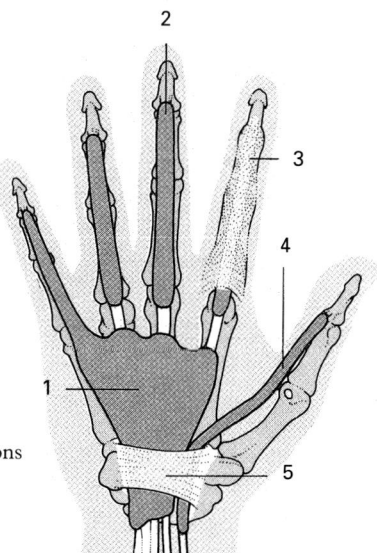

Answers on page 92   77

The Musculoskeletal System

Question 22
1. ____
2. ____
3. ____
4. ____
5. ____
6. ____
7. ____

A. Extensor pollicis brevis
B. Extensor retinaculum
C. Extensor carpi ulnaris
D. Extensor carpi radialis longus and brevis
E. Extensor digiti minimi
F. Extensor pollicis longus
G. Sheath for extensor digitorum

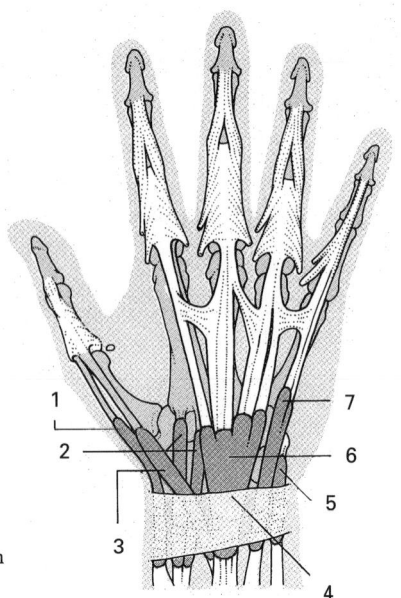

Question 23
1. ____
2. ____
3. ____
4. ____
5. ____
6. ____
7. ____
8. ____

A. Flexor digiti minimi
B. Flexor retinaculum
C. Adductor pollicis
D. Abductor pollicis brevis
E. Flexor pollicis brevis
F. Third lumbrical
G. Abductor digiti minimi
H. First lumbrical

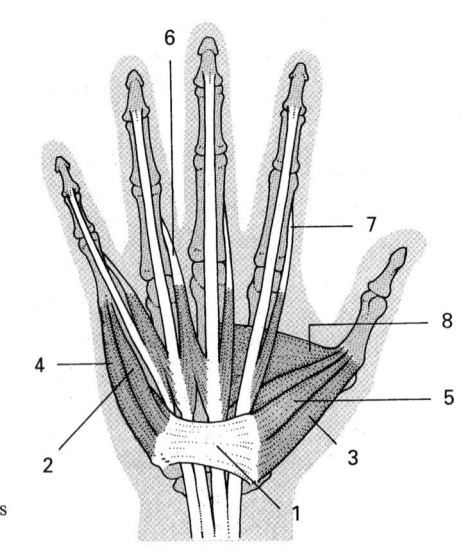

The Musculoskeletal System

Question 24

1. ____
2. ____

    A. Fourth palmar interosseus
    B. First palmar interosseus

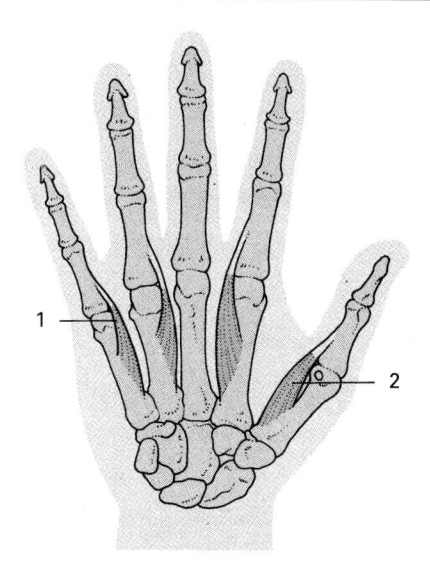

Question 25

1. ____
2. ____
3. ____
4. ____

    A. First dorsal interosseus
    B. Fourth dorsal interosseus
    C. Second dorsal interosseus
    D. Third dorsal interosseus

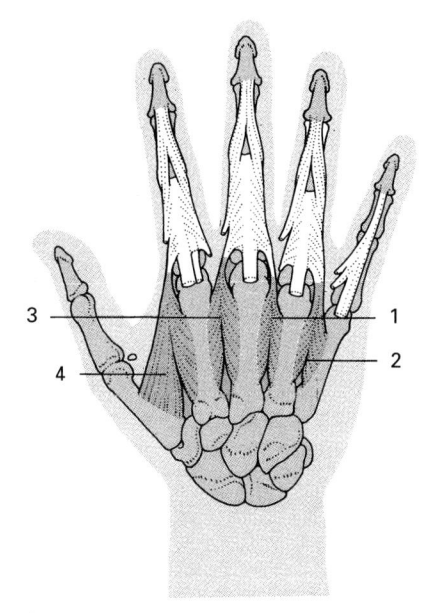

The Musculoskeletal System

Question 26

1. ____
2. ____
3. ____
4. ____
5. ____
6. ____
7. ____
8. ____
9. ____

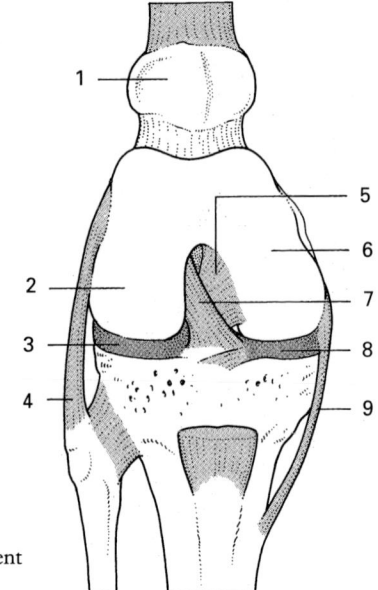

A. Lateral meniscus
B. Medial condyle
C. Medial meniscus
D. Patella
E. Medial (tibial) collateral ligament
F. Anterior cruciate ligament
G. Posterior cruciate ligament
H. Lateral condyle
I. Lateral (fibular) collateral ligament

The Musculoskeletal System

Question 27

1. ____
2. ____
3. ____
4. ____
5. ____
6. ____
7. ____
8. ____
9. ____
10. ____
11. ____
12. ____
13. ____
14. ____
15. ____
16. ____
17. ____
18. ____
19. ____
20. ____

A. Lateral patellar retinaculum
B. Lateral meniscus
C. Ligamentum patellae
D. Medial meniscus
E. Infrapatellar pad of fat
F. Posterior cruciate ligament
G. Popliteal artery and vein
H. Semitendinosus
I. Semimembranosus
J. Transverse ligament
K. Sartorius
L. Gracilis
M. Anterior cruciate ligament
N. Biceps
O. Tendon of popliteus
P. Medial patellar retinaculum
Q. Gastrocnemius (lateral head)
R. Lateral (fibular) collateral ligament
S. Tibial nerve
T. Gastrocnemius (medial head)

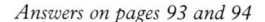

The Musculoskeletal System

Question 28
1. _____
2. _____
3. _____
4. _____
5. _____

A. Vastus lateralis
B. Sartorius
C. Rectus femoris
D. Vastus medialis
E. Vastus intermedius

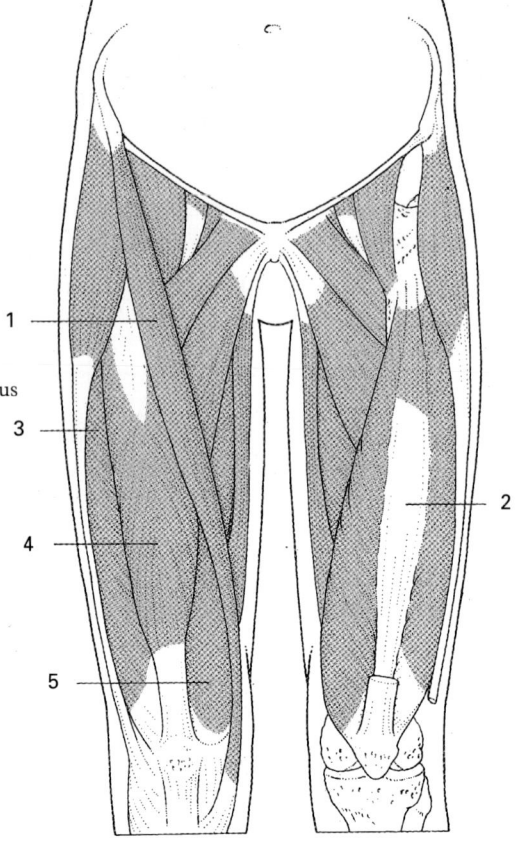

The Musculoskeletal System

Question 29
1. ____
2. ____
3. ____
4. ____
5. ____
6. ____
7. ____
8. ____

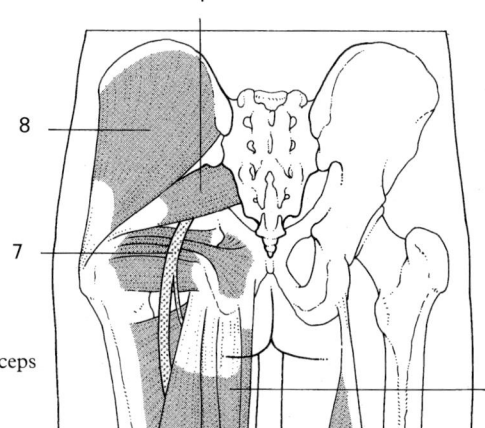

A. Short head of biceps
B. Semitendinosus
C. Biceps femoris
D. Gluteus medius
E. Adductor magnus
F. Piriformis
G. Semimembranosus
H. Sciatic nerve

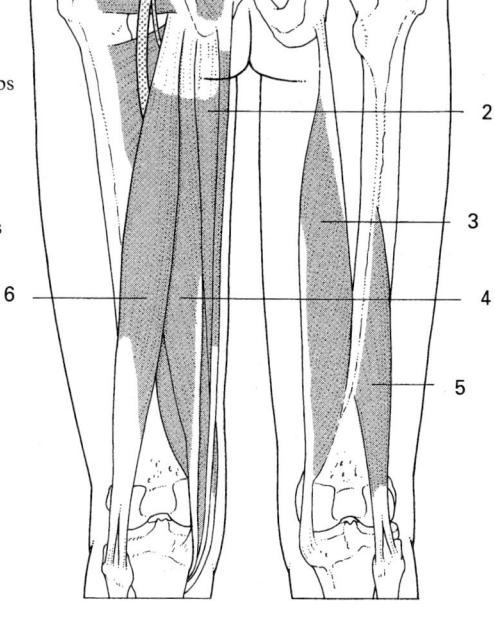

Answers on page 94

The Musculoskeletal System

Question 30

1. ____
2. ____
3. ____
4. ____
5. ____
6. ____

A. Tibialis anterior
B. Extensor digitorum longus
C. Extensor digitorum brevis
D. Extensor hallucis longus
E. Gastrocnemius
F. Soleus

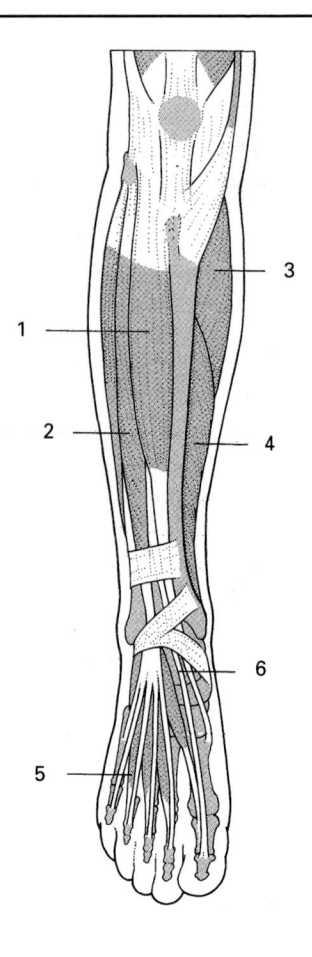

The Musculoskeletal System

Question 31
1. ____
2. ____
3. ____
4. ____
5. ____
6. ____
7. ____

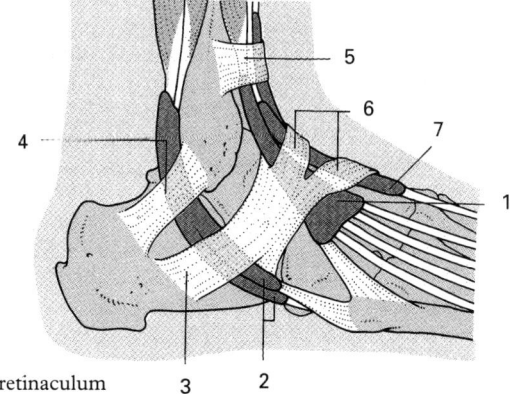

A. Inferior extensor retinaculum
B. Synovial sheath of extensor hallucis longus
C. Sheath of extensor digitorum longus
D. Peroneus longus and brevis (with synovial sheath)
E. Superior peroneal retinaculum
F. Inferior peroneal retinaculum
G. Superior extensor retinaculum

Question 32
1. ____
2. ____
3. ____
4. ____
5. ____
6. ____
7. ____

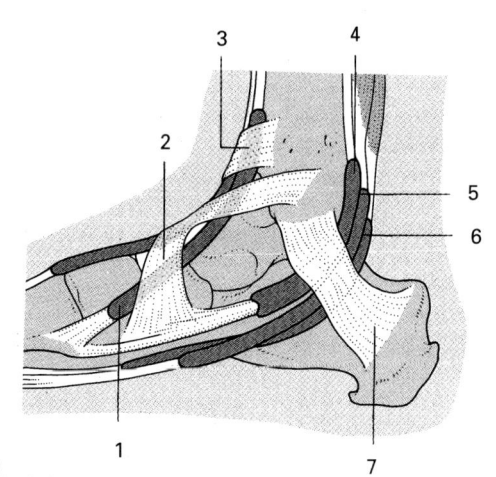

A. Flexor retinaculum
B. Sheath of flexor hallucis longus
C. Sheath of tibialis posterior
D. Synovial sheath of tibialis anterior
E. Sheath of flexor digitorum longus
F. Superior extensor retinaculum
G. Inferior extensor retinaculum

The Musculoskeletal System

A Picture questions

Question 1(i)
1. **D** Anterior arch
2. **C** Superior articular facet
3. **B** Transverse process
4. **A** Foramen transversarium
5. **E** Synovial joint for dens
6. **F** Posterior arch

Question 1(ii)
1. **E** Superior articular facet
2. **A** Dens
3. **C** Foramen transversarium
4. **D** Transverse process
5. **B** Spinous process

Question 2
1. **C** Costotransverse joint
2. **B** Costovertebral joint
3. **A** Superior articular facet

Question 3
1. **C** Costovertebral joint
2. **D** Superior articular facet
3. **E** Costotransverse joint
4. **B** Inferior articular facet
5. **A** Costovertebral joint

Question 4
1. **C** Annulus fibrosus
2. **A** Nucleus pulposus
3. **D** Hyaline cartilage
4. **F** Facet joint
5. **E** Inferior articular facet
6. **B** Intervertebral foramen
7. **G** Intervertebral disc

The Musculoskeletal System

Question 5
1. **B** Body of L3
2. **E** Rib 12
3. **C** Intervertebral foramen for 2nd lumbar spinal nerve
4. **F** L4 spinous process
5. **A** L4/L5 facet joint
6. **D** L4/L5 disc space

Question 6
1. **A** Internal auditory meatus
2. **I** Arcuate eminence
3. **B** Squamous part of temporal bone
4. **H** Tegmen tympani
5. **C** Foramen spinosum
6. **G** Posterior clinoid process
7. **D** Anterior clinoid process
8. **E** Optic canal
9. **F** Orbital plate of frontal bone
10. **N** Cribriform plate
11. **O** Crista galli
12. **S** Petrous part of temporal bone
13. **K** Foramen lacerum
14. **J** Middle cranial fossa
15. **R** Foramen ovale
16. **Q** Hypophyseal fossa
17. **W** Foramen rotundum
18. **P** Greater wing of sphenoid
19. **U** Lesser wing of sphenoid
20. **T** Posterior cranial fossa
21. **M** Internal occipital protruberance
22. **L** Foramen magnum
23. **V** Anterior cranial fossa

The Musculoskeletal System

Question 7
1. **B** Alveolar process
2. **D** Zygomatic arch
3. **R** Carotid canal
4. **H** Pharyngeal tubercle
5. **C** Jugular foramen
6. **G** Stylomastoid foramen
7. **I** Groove for digastric muscle
8. **Q** Incisor foramen
9. **F** Palatal process of maxilla
10. **E** Horizontal plate of palatine bone
11. **M** Greater palatine foramen
12. **S** Medial pterygoid plate
13. **L** Lateral pterygoid plate
14. **K** Foramen ovale
15. **J** Foramen spinosum
16. **T** Styloid process
17. **N** Occipital condyle
18. **P** Mastoid process
19. **O** Foramen magnum
20. **A** Inferior nuchal line

Question 8
1. **C** Lesser wing of sphenoid
2. **A** Lambdoid suture
3. **F** Frontal sinus
4. **H** Ethmoidal sinuses
5. **G** Maxillary sinus
6. **D** Fillings in teeth
7. **I** Inferior concha
8. **E** Nasal septum
9. **B** Supraorbital fissure

The Musculoskeletal System

Question 9
1. D Petrous temporal bone
2. F Mastoid air cells
3. E Grooves for middle meningeal vessels
4. H Top of the ear
5. I Posterior clinoid process
6. K Hypophyseal fossa
7. J Sphenoid air sinus
8. G Maxillary sinus
9. C Fillings in teeth
10. B Odontoid process of axis
11. A Posterior arch of atlas

Question 10
1. A Rectus capitis lateralis
2. B Rectus capitis anterior
3. D Longus capitis
4. G Longus colli
5. H Brachial plexus
6. I Scalenus medius
7. E Scalenus anterior
8. F Subclavian artery
9. C Apical pleura

Question 11
1. A Intercostal artery
2. E Intercostal nerve
3. B Internal intercostals
4. D External intercostals
5. C Intercostal vein

The Musculoskeletal System

A Question 12
1. **H** Rectus abdominis
2. **B** Transversalis fascia
3. **K** Rectus abdominis
4. **O** Transversalis fascia
5. **A** Lumbar vertebra
6. **G** Psoas major
7. **F** Quadratus lumborum
8. **N** Erector spinae
9. **M** Lumbar fascia
10. **L** Transversus abdominis
11. **I** Internal oblique
12. **J** External oblique
13. **E** External oblique
14. **D** Internal oblique
15. **C** Transversus abdominis

Question 13
1. **D** Internal oblique
2. **B** External oblique
3. **A** Inguinal ligament
4. **C** Rectus abdominis

Question 14
1. **D** Inferior epigastric artery
2. **A** Obliterated umbilical artery
3. **G** Peritoneum
4. **I** Transversalis fascia
5. **H** Rectus abdominis
6. **J** Internal oblique and transversus abdominis (fused together)
7. **O** External oblique aponeurosis
8. **P** Testis
9. **Q** Tunica vaginalis (derived from peritoneum)
10. **S** Internal spermatic fascia (from transversalis fascia)
11. **R** Cremaster
12. **F** External spermatic fascia
13. **L** Skin
14. **M** Subcutaneous fat
15. **N** External oblique
16. **K** Internal oblique
17. **E** Transversus abdominis
18. **B** Transversalis fascia
19. **C** Peritoneum

The Musculoskeletal System

Question 15
1. **E** Greater tuberosity (tubercle)
2. **F** Surgical neck
3. **H** Deltoid tuberosity
4. **G** Shaft
5. **K** Lateral supracondylar ridge
6. **N** Lateral epicondyle
7. **A** Capitulum
8. **B** Radial fossa
9. **O** Trochlea
10. **C** Medial epicondyle
11. **D** Coronoid fossa
12. **J** Bicipital groove
13. **M** Lesser tuberosity
14. **L** Head of humerus
15. **I** Anatomical neck
16. **Q** Spiral groove for radial nerve
17. **P** Lateral epicondyle
18. **T** Trochlea
19. **S** Olecranon fossa
20. **R** Medial epicondyle

Question 16
1. **B** Radial notch of ulna
2. **C** Trochlear notch
3. **E** Head of radius
4. **G** Coronoid process
5. **K** Radial tuberosity
6. **F** Head of ulna
7. **H** Styloid process of ulna
8. **A** Styloid process of radius
9. **J** Olecranon
10. **L** Styloid process of ulna
11. **D** Styloid process of radius
12. **I** Dorsal tubercle

The Musculoskeletal System

A
Question 17
1. **E** Ulna
2. **I** Lunate
3. **F** Triquetral
4. **L** Pisiform
5. **B** Capitate
6. **A** Hamate
7. **C** Trapezoid
8. **D** First metacarpal
9. **H** Trapezium
10. **G** Scaphoid
11. **K** Radial styloid process
12. **J** Radius

Question 18
1. **F** Latissimus dorsi
2. **E** Teres major
3. **C** Teres minor
4. **B** Infraspinatus
5. **A** Supraspinatus
6. **D** Deltoid

Question 19
1. **A** Flexor carpi ulnaris
2. **C** Palmaris longus
3. **B** Flexor carpi radialis
4. **E** Brachioradialis
5. **D** Pronator teres

Question 20
1. **A** Fibrous flexor sheath
2. **D** Dorsal interosseus
3. **C** Flexor digitorum superficialis
4. **B** Flexor digitorum profundus

Question 21
1. **C** Synovial sheath for flexor tendons
2. **E** Synovial sheath for flexor tendons to middle finger
3. **A** Fibrous flexor sheath
4. **D** Synovial sheath for flexor pollicis longus
5. **B** Flexor retinaculum

The Musculoskeletal System

Question 22
1. **A** Extensor pollicis brevis
2. **D** Extensor carpi radialis longus and brevis
3. **F** Extensor pollicis longus
4. **B** Extensor retinaculum
5. **C** Extensor carpi ulnaris
6. **G** Sheath for extensor digitorum
7. **E** Extensor digiti minimi

Question 23
1. **B** Flexor retinaculum
2. **A** Flexor digiti minimi
3. **D** Abductor pollicis brevis
4. **G** Abductor digiti minimi
5. **E** Flexor pollicis brevis
6. **F** Third lumbrical
7. **H** First lumbrical
8. **C** Adductor pollicis

Question 24
1. **A** Fourth palmar interosseus
2. **B** First palmar interosseus

Question 25
1. **D** Third dorsal interosseus
2. **B** Fourth dorsal interosseus
3. **C** Second dorsal interosseus
4. **A** First dorsal interosseus

Question 26
1. **D** Patella
2. **H** Lateral condyle
3. **A** Lateral meniscus
4. **I** Lateral (fibular) collateral ligament
5. **G** Posterior cruciate ligament
6. **B** Medial condyle
7. **F** Anterior cruciate ligament
8. **C** Medial meniscus
9. **E** Medial (tibial) collateral ligament

The Musculoskeletal System

Question 27
1. **C** Ligamentum patellae
2. **E** Infrapatellar pad of fat
3. **J** Transverse ligament
4. **P** Medial patellar retinaculum
5. **D** Medial meniscus
6. **K** Sartorius
7. **L** Gracilis
8. **H** Semitendinosus
9. **I** Semimembranosus
10. **T** Gastrocnemius (medial head)
11. **S** Tibial nerve
12. **G** Popliteal artery and vein
13. **Q** Gastrocnemius (lateral head)
14. **N** Biceps
15. **O** Tendon of popliteus
16. **R** Lateral (fibular) collateral ligament
17. **B** Lateral meniscus
18. **F** Posterior cruciate ligament
19. **M** Anterior cruciate ligament
20. **A** Lateral patellar retinaculum

Question 28
1. **B** Sartorius
2. **E** Vastus intermedius
3. **A** Vastus lateralis
4. **C** Rectus femoris
5. **D** Vastus medialis

Question 29
1. **F** Piriformis
2. **E** Adductor magnus
3. **G** Semimembranosus
4. **B** Semitendinosus
5. **A** Short head of biceps
6. **C** Biceps femoris
7. **H** Sciatic nerve
8. **D** Gluteus medius

The Musculoskeletal System

Question 30
1. **A** Tibialis anterior
2. **B** Extensor digitorum longus
3. **E** Gastrocnemius
4. **F** Soleus
5. **C** Extensor digitorum brevis
6. **D** Extensor hallucis longus

Question 31
1. **C** Sheath of extensor digitorum longus
2. **D** Peroneus longus and brevis (with synovial sheath)
3. **F** Inferior peroneal retinaculum
4. **E** Superior peroneal retinaculum
5. **G** Superior extensor retinaculum
6. **A** Inferior extensor retinaculum
7. **B** Synovial sheath of extensor hallucis longus

Question 32
1. **D** Synovial sheath of tibialis anterior
2. **G** Inferior extensor retinaculum
3. **F** Superior extensor retinaculum
4. **C** Sheath of tibialis posterior
5. **E** Sheath of flexor digitorum longus
6. **B** Sheath of flexor hallucis longus
7. **A** Flexor retinaculum

The Musculoskeletal System

Clinical problems

1. A 43-year-old college professor tried to push his car which was caught in a snowdrift, and suffered a severe pain in the lower back. He felt as if something had snapped in the lower part of his spine. He was later diagnosed as having a prolapse of the intervertebral disc between L5 and S1 vertebrae. What nerve root is most likely to be compressed by this injury and what may be your findings on examination of the patient?

2. A 20-year-old college student twisted his right knee while playing football and injured one of his menisci. Which meniscus is more likely to be damaged and why?

3. Why is the shoulder joint prone to dislocation? What factors normally stabilise the joint?

4. Following a subtrochanteric fracture of the femur, the proximal fragment may be flexed and abducted and the distal fragment may be pulled upwards, shortening the limb. Which muscles are responsible for these deformities?

5. A 60-year-old lady was brought to the Accident and Emergency Department following a fall on her outstretched hand. She was diagnosed as having a Colles' fracture and the appropriate treatment was given. At a later date she consulted her doctor complaining that she was unable to straighten the terminal phalanx of her thumb on the side of the fracture. What might have caused this problem? How can this be treated?

Answers on page 98

The Musculoskeletal System

A Clinical problems

1. A prolapse (herniation) of the nucleus pulposus of the L5/S1 disc is most likely to have compressed the S1 nerve root. This will result in pain on straight-leg raising due to stretching of the sciatic nerve. The patient may have weakness of his plantar flexors and the ankle jerk (S1, S2) will be weak. Sensory loss is variable and may be confined to the lateral border of the foot.

2. The medial meniscus is more likely to have been damaged as it is attached to the medial collateral ligament. When the knee is twisted, the collateral ligament is taut and it fixes the meniscus which gets trapped between the extending femur and tibia. The lateral meniscus is not attached to the lateral collateral ligament. This, together with the fact that the popliteus muscle is attached to it, makes the lateral meniscus more mobile than the medial meniscus.

3. Mobility of the shoulder joint is achieved at the expense of stability. The disproportionately large head of the humerus relative to the glenoid cavity, a lax and thin capsule, and the paucity of thick strong ligaments make the shoulder very mobile but relatively unstable. The tendons of the rotator cuff muscles fusing with the capsule, the coraco-acromial arch formed by the coraco-acromial ligament and the acromion preventing upward displacement, the glenoid labrum deepening the socket, and the long head of biceps passing through the joint winding over the head of the humerus are the main factors stabilising the shoulder joint.

4. The proximal fragment is flexed by the psoas major and abducted by the gluteus medius and minimus. The distal fragment may be displaced upwards by the pull of the adductors attached to the shaft of the femur.

5. This condition is called a 'mallet thumb' and is caused by rupture of the extensor pollicis longus tendon. It can happen following a Colles' fracture. The distal phalanx is kept flexed by the action of flexor pollicis longus and can only be extended passively. It can be treated by attaching the cut end of the tendon to extensor indicis, extensor carpi radialis longus or extensor pollicis brevis.

The Nervous System

The Nervous System

THE NERVOUS SYSTEM

True/False

1. **The cerebellum and cerebral hemispheres are separated by**
   a) the falx cerebri
   b) the tentorium cerebelli
   c) the diaphragma sellae
   d) the galea aponeurotica
   e) the falx cerebelli

2. **The following structures are developed from the hindbrain:**
   a) cerebellum
   b) lamina terminalis
   c) corpora quadrigemina
   d) medulla oblongata
   e) hypothalamus

3. **The hypothalamus**
   a) is part of the hindbrain
   b) forms the lateral wall of the third ventricle
   c) lies behind the thalamus
   d) controls endocrine functions
   e) is connected to the posterior lobe of the pituitary

4. **With regard to the midbrain:**
   a) the cerebral peduncles lie posteriorly
   b) the superior colliculi are concerned with auditory reflexes
   c) it is closely related to the free border of the falx cerebri
   d) the fourth cranial nerve takes origin from the upper part
   e) it contains the cerebral aqueduct

The Nervous System

1. a) **FALSE** The falx cerebri lies between the two cerebral hemispheres.
   b) **TRUE** The tentorium is attached to the petrous temporal bone.
   c) **FALSE** The diaphragma sellae roofs the pituitary fossa.
   d) **FALSE** This is part of the scalp.
   e) **FALSE** The falx cerebelli lies below the tentorium cerebelli in the median plane and projects into the posterior cerebellar notch.

2. a) **TRUE**
   b) **FALSE** This is the cranial end of the neural tube.
   c) **FALSE** These are parts of the midbrain.
   d) **TRUE** It lies below the pons.
   e) **FALSE**

3. a) **FALSE** It is part of the diencephalon (middle portion of the forebrain).
   b) **TRUE** The third ventricle also lies between the two thalami.
   c) **FALSE** The hypothalamus lies in front of the thalamus, separated from it by the hypothalamic sulcus.
   d) **TRUE**
   e) **TRUE** Hormones produced by the hypothalamus are transported to the posterior pituitary through the neuronal connections.

4. a) **FALSE** They form the anterior part of the midbrain.
   b) **FALSE** They are concerned with visual reflexes.
   c) **TRUE**
   d) **FALSE** It is the third cranial nerve (oculomotor) that originates from the upper part. The fourth nerve (trochlear) arises from the lower part.
   e) **TRUE** It connects the third and fourth ventricles.

The Nervous System

5. **The lateral ventricle**
   a) is the cavity of the midbrain
   b) opens into the third ventricle by the cerebral aqueduct
   c) is roofed by the corpus callosum
   d) extends into the temporal lobe
   e) does not produce cerebrospinal fluid

6. **The third ventricle**
   a) is part of the midbrain
   b) lies between the two thalami and the two hypothalami
   c) communicates with the fourth ventricle by the cerebral aqueduct
   d) is related to the pineal gland
   e) does not produce cerebrospinal fluid

7. **With regard to the fourth ventricle:**
   a) it lies in the hindbrain
   b) the posterior aspect of the pons and medulla form the anterior wall
   c) the abducens nerve is in its roof
   d) it communicates with the subarachnoid space by a single aperture
   e) it does not produce cerebrospinal fluid

8. **The following arteries form the circle of Willis:**
   a) middle cerebral artery
   b) anterior cerebral arteries
   c) anterior communicating artery
   d) posterior communicating artery
   e) posterior cerebral arteries

The Nervous System

5. a) **FALSE** It is the cavity of the telencephalon part of the forebrain.
    b) **FALSE** The interventricular foramen (of Monroe) is the connection with the third ventricle.
    c) **TRUE**
    d) **TRUE** This is its inferior horn.
    e) **FALSE** There are choroid plexuses in both the body and the inferior horn of the lateral ventricle.

6. a) **FALSE** It is the cavity of the diencephalon part of the forebrain.
    b) **TRUE**
    c) **TRUE**
    d) **TRUE** The pineal gland lies posteriorly in the midline.
    e) **FALSE** There are choroid plexuses hanging from the roof of the third ventricle.

7. a) **TRUE** It is the cavity of the hindbrain.
    b) **TRUE**
    c) **FALSE** The abducens nerve with the facial nerve winding around it forms the facial colliculus on the floor of the fourth ventricle.
    d) **FALSE** There are three apertures, one in the midline (foramen of Magendie) and two lateral (foramen of Luschka).
    e) **FALSE** There are choroid plexuses on the roof.

8. a) **FALSE** The internal carotid artery contributes to it.
    b) **TRUE** These are branches of the internal carotid artery.
    c) **TRUE** It connects the two anterior cerebral arteries.
    d) **TRUE** It connects the internal carotid artery to the posterior cerebral artery.
    e) **TRUE**

The Nervous System

9. **The posterior cerebral artery**
   a) is a branch of the internal carotid artery
   b) is closely related to the oculomotor nerve
   c) supplies the visual cortex
   d) if occluded unilaterally, causes bitemporal hemianopia
   e) is connected to the internal carotid artery by the posterior communicating artery

10. **Concerning the venous drainage of the brain:**
    a) the anterior cerebral vein drains into the basal vein
    b) the basal vein drains into the great cerebral vein of Galen
    c) there are commonly six superior cerebral veins
    d) the deep middle cerebral vein drains into the cavernous sinus
    e) these veins have no valves

11. **The sigmoid sinus**
    a) is a direct continuation of the straight sinus
    b) grooves the sphenoid bone
    c) ends at the jugular foramen
    d) is closely related to the mastoid antrum
    e) receives blood from the cavernous sinus

12. **The cranial venous sinuses**
    a) lie between the dura and pia mater
    b) form the main venous drainage of the brain
    c) communicate with extracranial veins
    d) can be involved in acute mastoiditis
    e) all drain to the superior sagittal sinus

The Nervous System

9. a) **FALSE** It is a branch of the basilar artery; the latter is formed by the two vertebral arteries.
    b) **TRUE** The nerve lies between the posterior cerebral and the superior cerebellar arteries.
    c) **TRUE**
    d) **FALSE** It causes homonymus hemianopia.
    e) **TRUE**

10. a) **TRUE** The anterior cerebral vein accompanies the corresponding artery.
    b) **TRUE** The great cerebral vein is formed by the union of the two internal cerebral veins.
    c) **FALSE** There are usually about 8–12.
    d) **FALSE** The superficial middle cerebral vein drains into the cavernous sinus. The deep vein drains into the basal vein.
    e) **TRUE**

11. a) **FALSE** It is a continuation of the transverse sinus.
    b) **FALSE** It grooves the occipital bone.
    c) **FALSE** It ends below the jugular foramen.
    d) **TRUE**
    e) **TRUE** Through the superior and inferior petrosal sinuses.

12. a) **FALSE** They lie within the dura mater.
    b) **TRUE**
    c) **TRUE** Through emissary veins.
    d) **TRUE**
    e) **FALSE**

The Nervous System

13. **With regard to the cavernous sinus:**
    a) it is related medially to the pituitary gland
    b) infection from the face can reach the sinus through the pterygoid plexus of veins
    c) the ophthalmic artery passes through the sinus
    d) the abducens nerve accompanies the internal carotid artery
    e) the mandibular nerve lies on the lateral wall

14. **The following are connected to the cavernous sinus:**
    a) ophthalmic veins
    b) superficial middle cerebral vein
    c) superior petrosal sinus
    d) inferior petrosal sinus
    e) middle meningeal vein

15. **The middle meningeal artery**
    a) lies in the subarachnoid space
    b) lies in the subdural space
    c) lies in the extradural space
    d) is a branch of the maxillary artery
    e) enters the skull through the foramen spinosum

16. **The subarachnoid space**
    a) contains the cerebral vessels
    b) contains the cerebrospinal fluid
    c) extends down to the lower end of the spinal cord at the level of L1
    d) extends along the whole length of the optic nerve
    e) lies between the pia and the arachnoid mater

The Nervous System

13. a) **TRUE**
    b) **TRUE** The cavernous sinus is connected inferiorly to the pterygoid plexus through emissary veins.
    c) **FALSE** The internal carotid artery passes through the sinus, and then gives off the ophthalmic artery.
    d) **TRUE**
    e) **FALSE** The maxillary and ophthalmic nerves lie on the lateral wall along with the oculomotor and trochlear nerves.

14. a) **TRUE**
    b) **TRUE**
    c) **TRUE** It connects the cavernous sinus to the transverse sinus.
    d) **TRUE** It connects the cavernous sinus to the internal jugular vein.
    e) **FALSE**

15. a) **FALSE**
    b) **FALSE**
    c) **TRUE**
    d) **TRUE**
    e) **TRUE**

16. a) **TRUE**
    b) **TRUE**
    c) **FALSE** It extends beyond the spinal cord, to the lower border of the second sacral vertebra.
    d) **TRUE**
    e) **TRUE**

The Nervous System

17. **The subdural space**
    a) contains choroid plexus
    b) contains cerebral veins before they drain into the dural venous sinuses
    c) contains meningeal vessels
    d) contains cerebrospinal fluid
    e) is replaced by the epidural space around the spinal cord

18. **Light passes through the following before reaching the retina:**
    a) the cornea
    b) the anterior chamber
    c) the posterior chamber
    d) the lens
    e) the vitreous chamber

19. **With regard to the retina:**
    a) it has two layers
    b) the optic disc lies lateral to the macula lutea
    c) the optic disc only has cones as photoreceptors
    d) the rods and cones lie towards the outer aspect
    e) its entire blood supply comes from the central artery of the retina

20. **Concerning the accommodation reflex (looking at a near object):**
    a) the suspensory ligaments tighten
    b) the pupils dilate
    c) the eyes converge
    d) it is abolished in a complete lesion of the oculomotor nerve
    e) the light reflex will be abolished and the accommodation reflex will be present in lesions of the pretectal nuclei

The Nervous System

17. a) **FALSE**
    b) **TRUE**
    c) **FALSE** These are extradural.
    d) **FALSE**
    e) **FALSE**

18. a) **TRUE**
    b) **TRUE** This lies between the iris and the cornea.
    c) **TRUE** This lies behind the iris and pupil and communicates with the anterior chamber through the pupil.
    d) **TRUE**
    e) **TRUE**

19. a) **TRUE** The retina has an inner and an outer layer. The inner layer contains the pars optica retina, which is multilayered and generates visual impulses.
    b) **FALSE** The disc lies medial to the macula.
    c) **FALSE** The disc is the commencement of the optic nerve and has no photoreceptor. The fovea centralis in the macula possesses only cones.
    d) **TRUE** Hence light rays pass through the whole thickness of the retina (i.e. the pars optica retina) to stimulate them.
    e) **TRUE** This is a branch of the ophthalmic artery (derived from the internal carotid) and does not anastomose with any other artery.

20. a) **FALSE** They slacken by contraction of the ciliary muscles, making the lens bulge more.
    b) **FALSE** They constrict.
    c) **TRUE**
    d) **TRUE**
    e) **TRUE** This is known as the Argyll-Robertson pupil.

The Nervous System

21. The following statements about the visual pathway are true:
   a) the posterior cerebellar artery supplies it
   b) fibres synapse in the medial geniculate body
   c) a lesion of the central part of the optic chiasma causes nasal hemianopia
   d) the visual centre is on the calcarine sulcus
   e) the inferior corpora quadrigemina (inferior colliculi) are visual relay stations

22. With regard to the middle ear:
   a) the aditus opens from its posterior wall
   b) it develops from the first pharyngeal pouch
   c) the seventh cranial nerve runs on the upper part of the medial wall
   d) the auditory tube opens into its posterior wall
   e) it is supplied by the auriculotemporal nerve

23. With regard to the ossicles of the middle ear:
   a) the stapes articulates with the malleus
   b) the handle of the malleus is attached to the tympanic membrane
   c) the chorda tympani crosses the tympanic membrane
   d) stapedius is attached to the handle of the malleus
   e) the malleus is derived from the first branchial arch

24. Concerning the mastoid:
   a) it is a part of the occipital bone
   b) the mastoid antrum is fully developed at birth
   c) the mastoid air cells are fully developed at birth
   d) the antrum is connected to the middle ear
   e) the antrum and the air cells are closely related to the cavernous sinus

The Nervous System

21. a) **FALSE** It is the posterior cerebral artery that supplies it.
    b) **FALSE** Fibres synapse in the lateral geniculate body.
    c) **FALSE** This causes bitemporal hemianopia.
    d) **TRUE** The calcarine sulcus lies on the medial aspect of the occipital lobe.
    e) **FALSE** The superior corpora quadrigemina (superior colliculi) are visual relay stations.

22. a) **TRUE** It connects the middle ear to the mastoid antrum.
    b) **TRUE** The middle ear, mastoid antrum and auditory tube are derived from the first pouch.
    c) **TRUE** The nerve lies in its own canal.
    d) **FALSE** It opens on the anterior wall.
    e) **FALSE** It is supplied by the glossopharyngeal nerve.

23. a) **FALSE** The incus articulates with the malleus, and the stapes with the incus.
    b) **TRUE** The tympanic membrane separates the middle ear from the external auditory meatus.
    c) **TRUE** The nerve lies on the inner aspect of the membrane.
    d) **FALSE** It is attached to the stapes; tensor tympani is attached to the malleus.
    e) **TRUE** As is the incus; the stapes is derived from the second arch.

24. a) **FALSE** It is a part of the temporal bone.
    b) **TRUE**
    c) **FALSE**
    d) **TRUE** By the aditus.
    e) **FALSE** They are closely related to the sigmoid sinus.

The Nervous System

25. **The following cranial nerves carry parasympathetic fibres:**
    a) facial
    b) ophthalmic
    c) ninth (glossopharyngeal)
    d) sixth (abducens)
    e) third (oculomotor)

26. **With regard to the oculomotor nerve:**
    a) it emerges from the midbrain
    b) it may be damaged, resulting in ptosis
    c) it contains preganglionic parasympathetic fibres
    d) it carries motor fibres to all the extrinsic eye muscles except the superior oblique
    e) paralysis causes medial deviation of the eye

27. **The oculomotor nerve supplies**
    a) the ciliary muscle
    b) the superior oblique muscle
    c) the inferior oblique muscle
    d) the conjunctiva
    e) the dilator pupillae muscle

28. **The trigeminal nerve**
    a) has a small motor and a large sensory root
    b) includes the nasal cavity in its sensory distribution
    c) emerges from the lateral part of the pons
    d) has a ganglion in the posterior cranial fossa
    e) has a motor root that goes through the ganglion

29. **The trigeminal nerve has branches traversing**
    a) the foramen rotundum
    b) the superior orbital fissure
    c) the foramen ovale
    d) the foramen lacerum
    e) the optic canal

The Nervous System

25. a) TRUE
    b) FALSE
    c) TRUE
    d) FALSE
    e) TRUE

26. a) TRUE
    b) TRUE   It supplies the levator palpebrae superioris muscle.
    c) TRUE   These are from the Edinger-Westphal nucleus. They synapse in the ciliary ganglion. Postganglionic fibres supply the constrictor pupillae and ciliary muscles.
    d) FALSE It supplies motor fibres to all the extrinsic eye muscles except superior oblique (IV nerve) and lateral rectus (VI nerve).
    e) FALSE The eye deviates laterally.

27. a) TRUE
    b) FALSE
    c) TRUE
    d) FALSE The conjunctiva is supplied by the trigeminal nerve.
    e) FALSE This is supplied by the sympathetic nerves.

28. a) TRUE
    b) TRUE
    c) TRUE
    d) FALSE Its ganglion is in the middle cranial fossa, in the Meckel's cave.
    e) FALSE It lies under the ganglion.

29. a) TRUE   Maxillary nerve.
    b) TRUE   Ophthalmic nerve.
    c) TRUE   Mandibular nerve.
    d) FALSE This contains the internal carotid artery.
    e) FALSE The optic canal contains the optic nerve and the ophthalmic artery.

The Nervous System

30. **The fifth cranial nerve**
    a) arises from the pons
    b) is the motor nerve to the muscles of mastication
    c) is sensory to the face
    d) provides a sensory and a motor root to the semilunar ganglion
    e) has a nucleus that forms the facial colliculus

31. **The cervical sympathetic trunk**
    a) lies anterior to scalenus anterior
    b) is enclosed in the carotid sheath
    c) has three cardiac branches
    d) gives off a branch to the pharyngeal plexus
    e) receives preganglionic fibres from T1 and T2

32. **The cervicothoracic (stellate) ganglion**
    a) lies anterior to the neck of the first rib
    b) lies medial to the superior intercostal artery
    c) lies anterior to the vertebral artery
    d) supplies branches to the axillary artery
    e) supplies branches to the vertebral artery

33. **Fibres from the following synapse on cells of the submandibular ganglion:**
    a) fifth cranial nerve
    b) chorda tympani
    c) sympathetic fibres from the superior cervical ganglion
    d) twelfth cranial nerve
    e) lingual nerve

The Nervous System

30. a) **TRUE**
b) **TRUE**
c) **TRUE**
d) **FALSE** Only the sensory root is attached to the ganglion.
e) **FALSE**

31. a) **FALSE** It is more medial and lies just posterior to the carotid sheath.
b) **FALSE**
c) **TRUE** Each cervical ganglion gives off a cardiac branch.
d) **TRUE**
e) **TRUE**

32. a) **TRUE**
b) **TRUE**
c) **FALSE** It lies posterior to the artery.
d) **TRUE**
e) **TRUE**

33. a) **FALSE**
b) **TRUE**
c) **FALSE**
d) **FALSE**
e) **FALSE**

115

The Nervous System

34. The ciliary ganglion
   a) receives sensory fibres from the seventh cranial nerve ____
   b) receives sympathetic fibres from the internal carotid plexus ____
   c) receives parasympathetic fibres from the oculomotor nerve ____
   d) controls eye movement ____
   e) is enclosed in a prolongation of dura mater ____

35. The sixth nerve
   a) supplies the superior oblique muscle ____
   b) supplies the medial rectus muscle ____
   c) supplies muscles which direct the eyeball laterally ____
   d) leaves the brainstem between the olive and the pyramid ____
   e) has a nucleus that forms the facial colliculus ____

36. The twelfth nerve
   a) arises from the floor of the fourth ventricle ____
   b) passes through the jugular foramen ____
   c) lies superficial to the carotid arteries ____
   d) runs deep to hyoglossus ____
   e) supplies all the muscles of the tongue ____

37. The superior laryngeal nerve
   a) passes between the internal carotid artery and the external carotid artery ____
   b) has cells of origin at the medulla oblongata ____
   c) supplies the middle constrictor muscle ____
   d) gives a branch which lies in the submucosa of the piriform fossa ____
   e) is purely motor ____

The Nervous System

34. a) **FALSE** It receives sensory fibres from the nasociliary (ophthalmic) nerve.
    b) **TRUE**
    c) **TRUE**
    d) **FALSE** It controls the size of the pupil.
    e) **FALSE**

35. a) **FALSE** Superior oblique is supplied by the trochlear nerve.
    b) **FALSE** Medial rectus is supplied by the oculomotor nerve.
    c) **TRUE**
    d) **FALSE** It leaves the brainstem at the junction between the pons and medulla, near the midline.
    e) **TRUE** Together with the facial nerve fibres which wind round it.

36. a) **TRUE** It arises from the hypoglossal nucleus.
    b) **FALSE** It passes through the hypoglossal canal.
    c) **TRUE**
    d) **FALSE** It lies on hyoglossus.
    e) **FALSE** It supplies all the intrinsic and extrinsic muscles except palatoglossus.

37. a) **FALSE** It lies deep to the carotids.
    b) **TRUE** Its motor fibres originate from the nucleus ambiguus.
    c) **FALSE** It supplies the cricothyroid. All the constrictors are supplied by the pharyngeal branch of the vagus nerve.
    d) **TRUE** This is the internal laryngeal nerve.
    e) **FALSE** The internal laryngeal nerve is sensory.

The Nervous System

38. **The pharyngeal branch of the vagus**
    a) has fibres originating in the nucleus ambiguus
    b) lies between the internal and external carotids
    c) supplies all the muscles of the pharynx
    d) supplies muscles of the larynx
    e) supplies muscles of the soft palate

39. **The features of Horner's syndrome**
    a) are caused by paralysis of the cervical sympathetic trunk
    b) include dilation of the pupil
    c) include dry skin
    d) include exophthalmos
    e) include ptosis

40. **The lingual nerve as it lies on hyoglossus**
    a) is crossed by the submandibular duct
    b) carries taste fibres from the tongue
    c) supplies the vallate papillae
    d) carries motor function to the tongue
    e) carries parasympathetic nerves

41. **With regard to the facial nerve:**
    a) the temporal branch runs under the zygomatic arch
    b) it lies deep within the parotid gland
    c) it passes through the stylomastoid foramen
    d) if the upper part of the face is spared, the lesion is above the pons
    e) the lesser superficial petrosal nerve is one of its branches

The Nervous System

38. a) **TRUE**
b) **TRUE**
c) **FALSE** It supplies all the muscles of the pharynx except the stylopharyngeus (IX nerve).
d) **FALSE**
e) **TRUE** It supplies all the muscles except tensor palati (mandibular nerve).

39. a) **TRUE**
b) **FALSE** There is constriction of the pupil (dilator pupillae is supplied by sympathetics).
c) **TRUE** Due to the absence of sweating.
d) **FALSE** There may be slight enophthalmos.
e) **TRUE** The sympathetics supply part of the levator palpebrae superioris.

40. a) **TRUE**
b) **TRUE**
c) **FALSE** These are supplied by the glossopharyngeal nerve.
d) **FALSE**
e) **TRUE** They supply the submandibular and sublingual glands.

41. a) **FALSE** The nerve lies on the zygomatic arch.
b) **TRUE**
c) **TRUE**
d) **TRUE** This will be a supranuclear (upper motor neurone) paralysis. The nucleus lies in the pons.
e) **FALSE** The greater superficial petrosal is a branch.

The Nervous System

42. **The facial nerve**
    a) supplies the muscles of facial expression only
    b) supplies tensor tympani
    c) gives no sensory branches to the face
    d) is secretomotor to the nose, palate and lacrimal gland
    e) if sectioned, leads to an inability to close the eye

43. **The following are branches of the facial nerve:**
    a) auriculotemporal nerve
    b) nerve to stapedius
    c) chorda tympani
    d) nerve supply to levator anguli oris
    e) greater superficial petrosal nerve

44. **The facial nerve**
    a) supplies masseter
    b) supplies medial pterygoid
    c) supplies parasympathetic fibres to the lacrimal gland
    d) supplies buccinator
    e) supplies parasympathetic fibres to the parotid gland

45. **The chorda tympani carries**
    a) taste fibres for the anterior two-thirds of the tongue
    b) taste fibres for the posterior third of the tongue
    c) ordinary sensation for the anterior two-thirds of the tongue
    d) secretory fibres to the sublingual and submandibular glands
    e) cervical sympathetic fibres

The Nervous System

42. a) **FALSE** The facial nerve also supplies the posterior belly of digastric, stylohyoid and stapedius.
    b) **FALSE** It is supplied by the mandibular nerve.
    c) **TRUE**
    d) **TRUE** These fibres branch off as the greater petrosal nerve and synapse in the sphenopalatine ganglion.
    e) **TRUE** As the orbicularis oculi is supplied by the facial nerve.

43. a) **FALSE** This is a branch of the mandibular nerve.
    b) **TRUE** Paralysis causes hyperacusis.
    c) **TRUE** The chorda tympani carries taste and parasympathetic fibres.
    d) **TRUE** And the nerves supplying all the other muscles of facial expression.
    e) **TRUE**

44. a) **FALSE** Masseter is supplied by the mandibular nerve.
    b) **FALSE** Medial pterygoid is supplied by the mandibular nerve.
    c) **TRUE**
    d) **TRUE**
    e) **FALSE** The glossopharyngeal nerve does.

45. a) **TRUE**
    b) **FALSE** These are carried by the glossopharyngeal nerve.
    c) **FALSE** This is carried by the lingual nerve.
    d) **TRUE**
    e) **FALSE**

The Nervous System

46. **The following structures pass through the internal auditory meatus:**
    a) the nervus intermedius
    b) the auricular branch of the vagus
    c) the posterior inferior cerebellar artery
    d) the labyrinthine artery
    e) the eighth cranial nerve

47. **The inferior alveolar nerve**
    a) supplies mylohyoid
    b) supplies the skin of the cheek
    c) has a branch supplying the skin of the chin
    d) has a branch supplying the skin of the lower lip
    e) has a branch supplying the lower central incisor of the opposite side

48. **The phrenic nerve**
    a) carries fibres from C6–C8 spinal nerves
    b) has no afferent sensory fibres
    c) lies anterior to scalenus anterior
    d) lies anterior to the subclavian vein
    e) lies posterior to the root of the lung

49. **The phrenic nerve**
    a) lies in front of the prevertebral fascia on scalenus anterior
    b) is intimately related to the third part of the subclavian artery
    c) on the right side lies lateral to the right brachiocephalic vein
    d) supplies the crus of the diaphragm
    e) has its left nerve separated from the left vagus by the left superior intercostal vein

The Nervous System

46. a) **TRUE**
b) **FALSE**
c) **FALSE**
d) **TRUE**
e) **TRUE**

47. a) **TRUE** The nerve to mylohyoid branches off from it proximally (before entering the mandibular canal).
b) **FALSE** The skin of the cheek is supplied by the buccal nerve.
c) **TRUE** This is the mental nerve.
d) **TRUE** This is the mental nerve.
e) **TRUE** Branches of this nerve do not stop short at the midline.

48. a) **FALSE** From C3–C5 nerve roots.
b) **FALSE** It carries sensory fibres from the pericardium, pleura and peritoneum, and diaphragm.
c) **TRUE**
d) **FALSE** It lies posterior to the subclavian vein.
e) **FALSE** It is anterior to the root of the lung.

49. a) **FALSE** The phrenic nerve lies behind the prevertebral fascia.
b) **FALSE** It crosses the artery more medially.
c) **TRUE** It also lies lateral to the superior vena cava, right atrium and inferior vena cava.
d) **TRUE**
e) **TRUE**

The Nervous System

50. The left phrenic nerve
  a) supplies the right crus of the diaphragm
  b) lies posterior to scalenus anterior
  c) if paralysed will cause elevation of the diaphragm on the paralysed side
  d) carries afferent fibres from the pericardium
  e) carries afferent fibres from the lung

51. The following occur after section of the lower cervical part of the spinal cord:
  a) increased knee jerk
  b) loss of bladder function
  c) diaphragmatic breathing
  d) increased muscle tone
  e) loss of sensation on the medial part of the arm

52. Acute section of the spinal cord at the level of T1 causes
  a) paralysis of the ciliary muscle
  b) loss of sensation over the thumb
  c) paralysis of the small muscles of the hand
  d) loss of sensation in the neck
  e) loss of extension at the elbow

53. The spinal cord is supplied by
  a) the anterior spinal artery
  b) the posterior spinal artery
  c) the intercostal arteries
  d) the internal carotid artery
  e) the internal thoracic artery

The Nervous System

50. a) **TRUE** It supplies the part of the diaphragm to the left of the oesophagus and includes part of the right crus.
    b) **FALSE** It lies anterior to scalenus anterior.
    c) **TRUE**
    d) **TRUE**
    e) **FALSE** It carries afferents from the pleura.

51. a) **TRUE**
    b) **TRUE**
    c) **TRUE** The intercostal muscles will be paralysed.
    d) **TRUE**
    e) **TRUE**

52. a) **FALSE**
    b) **FALSE** This region is usually supplied by C6.
    c) **TRUE**
    d) **FALSE**
    e) **FALSE**

53. a) **TRUE** This is a branch of the vertebral artery.
    b) **TRUE** This is also a branch of the vertebral artery.
    c) **TRUE** These and the cervical and lumbar arteries from the aorta give radicular branches which reinforce the supply from the spinal arteries.
    d) **FALSE**
    e) **FALSE**

The Nervous System

54. The median nerve
   a) lies medial to the palmaris longus tendon at the wrist ____
   b) supplies the lateral part of the flexor digitorum profundus muscle by its anterior interosseous branch ____
   c) is derived from the posterior and medial cord of the brachial plexus ____
   d) supplies the skin over the distal phalanges of the index and middle fingers ____
   e) enters the forearm between the heads of the pronator teres muscle ____

55. Division of the long thoracic nerve is indicated by
   a) inability to retract the scapula ____
   b) wasting of the pectoralis major muscle ____
   c) weakness of adduction of the humerus ____
   d) winging of the scapula ____
   e) difficulty in pushing forward ____

56. The median nerve
   a) is derived from the medial and lateral cords of the brachial plexus ____
   b) contains T1 fibres ____
   c) supplies abductor pollicis brevis ____
   d) supplies the lateral two palmar interossei ____
   e) in the axilla lies medial to the axillary artery ____

57. The lateral cord of the brachial plexus
   a) contains motor fibres only ____
   b) gives rise to the musculocutaneous nerve ____
   c) may contribute to the ulnar nerve ____
   d) may be damaged in fractures of the surgical neck of the humerus ____
   e) contains T1 fibres ____

The Nervous System

54. a) **FALSE** It lies deep to the tendon, medial to the flexor carpi radialis.
   b) **TRUE**
   c) **FALSE** It is derived from the lateral and medial cords.
   d) **TRUE**
   e) **TRUE**

55. a) **FALSE** This will lead to inability to protract the scapula.
   b) **FALSE**
   c) **FALSE**
   d) **TRUE**
   e) **TRUE**

56. a) **TRUE**
   b) **TRUE**
   c) **TRUE**
   d) **FALSE** All the interossei are supplied by the ulnar nerve.
   e) **FALSE** The median nerve lies lateral to the artery at its commencement; it crosses to the medial side in the middle of the arm.

57. a) **FALSE** All the cords are mixed nerves.
   b) **TRUE**
   c) **TRUE** C7 fibres from the lateral cord may join the ulnar nerve anywhere during its course.
   d) **FALSE** The axillary nerve winds round the surgical neck.
   e) **FALSE** It contains C5, C6 and C7 fibres.

The Nervous System

58. A wrist lesion of the ulnar nerve results in
   a) inability to spread the fingers
   b) inability to oppose the thumb
   c) loss of sweating on the palmar aspect of the little finger
   d) inability to extend at the metacarpophalangeal joint
   e) loss of skin sensation over the hypothenar eminence

59. The radial nerve
   a) winds around the humerus
   b) runs part of its course in a groove between brachioradialis and brachialis
   c) occasionally supplies brachialis
   d) supplies the extensor carpi radialis longus muscle through its posterior interosseus branch
   e) supplies the dorsal interossei in the hand

60. The radial nerve
   a) is the only nerve of the posterior cord which reaches the forearm
   b) has root values C5 and C6
   c) has no area of cutaneous supply above the level of the elbow
   d) lies in contact with the humerus between the lateral and medial heads of triceps
   e) if damaged in the middle of the arm, leads to paralysis of triceps

61. Damage to the sciatic nerve results in
   a) loss of extension of the knee
   b) total loss of sensation below the knee
   c) loss of sensation on the sole of the foot
   d) inability to flex the hip
   e) loss of proprioception from the knee joint

The Nervous System

58. a) **TRUE** Due to paralysis of the dorsal interossei.
    b) **FALSE**
    c) **TRUE** Sympathetic fibres reach the skin through the nerve.
    d) **FALSE** Inability to flex the joint is due to paralysis of the lumbricals and interossei.
    e) **FALSE** This area is supplied by the palmar branch of the ulnar nerve which leaves the trunk higher up and hence escapes injury.

59. a) **TRUE** It lies in the radial groove.
    b) **TRUE**
    c) **TRUE** Brachialis is also supplied by the musculocutaneous nerve.
    d) **FALSE** This muscle is supplied by the trunk of the radial nerve in the lower part of the arm.
    e) **FALSE** All the interossei are supplied by the ulnar nerve.

60. a) **TRUE**
    b) **FALSE** The radial nerve has root values C5, C6, C7, C8 and T1.
    c) **FALSE** The posterior cutaneous nerve of the arm and the lower lateral cutaneous nerve of the arm are its branches.
    d) **TRUE** In the radial (spiral) groove.
    e) **FALSE** The branches to triceps are given off in the axilla.

61. a) **FALSE** The extensors of the knee (quadriceps) are supplied by the femoral nerve.
    b) **FALSE** The saphenous nerve (a branch of the femoral) supplies the medial part of the leg and foot.
    c) **TRUE** Due to paralysis of lateral and medial plantar nerves.
    d) **FALSE** The hip flexors are supplied by the branches of the lumbar plexus.
    e) **FALSE** The knee joint is also supplied by the obturator and the femoral nerves.

The Nervous System

62. **The sciatic nerve**
    a) divides into the common peroneal and tibial nerves at a variable level in the lower limb
    b) lies under cover of gluteus maximus midway between the greater trochanter and the ischial tuberosity
    c) is derived from the anterior rami of the L4, L5 and S1–S3 nerves
    d) supplies the gluteal muscles
    e) supplies the adductor magnus

63. **Destruction of the superior gluteal nerve may disturb the normal gait by paralysing**
    a) piriformis
    b) gluteus medius
    c) gluteus maximus
    d) hamstrings
    e) adductor magnus

64. **The inferior gluteal nerve supplies**
    a) gluteus minimus
    b) tensor fasciae latae
    c) gluteus medius
    d) gluteus maximus
    e) obturator externus

65. **A male patient has an aneurysm of the aorta extending across the left psoas muscle involving the genitofemoral nerve. This could produce**
    a) pain over the femoral triangle
    b) pain in the scrotum
    c) inability to elevate the testis
    d) inability to achieve erection
    e) inability to ejaculate

The Nervous System

62. a) **TRUE** The two divisions may remain separate as they come out of the pelvis.
    b) **TRUE** The nerve is also an important posterior relation of the hip joint.
    c) **TRUE** The anterior divisions contribute to the tibial nerve and the posterior divisions to the common peroneal.
    d) **FALSE** They are supplied by the superior and inferior gluteal nerves.
    e) **TRUE** This muscle is also supplied by the obturator nerve.

63. a) **FALSE** Piriformis is supplied by a branch directly from the sacral plexus.
    b) **TRUE**
    c) **FALSE** Gluteus maximus is supplied by the inferior gluteal nerve.
    d) **FALSE** Hamstrings are supplied by the sciatic nerve.
    e) **FALSE** Adductor magnus is supplied by the sciatic and the obturator nerve.

64. a) **FALSE** Gluteus minimus is supplied by the superior gluteal nerve.
    b) **FALSE** It is supplied by the superior gluteal nerve.
    c) **FALSE** It is supplied by the superior gluteal nerve.
    d) **TRUE**
    e) **FALSE** Obturator externus is supplied by the obturator nerve.

65. a) **TRUE** The femoral branch of the genitofemoral nerve supplies the skin over this area.
    b) **TRUE** The genital branch has some sensory fibres in the scrotum.
    c) **TRUE** The genital branch supplies the cremaster muscle.
    d) **FALSE** This is controlled by the parasympathetic nerves.
    e) **FALSE** Ejaculation is controlled by the sympathetic nerves.

The Nervous System

66. **Injury to the upper lateral margin of the popliteal fossa may damage the following nerves:**
    a) common peroneal _____
    b) tibial _____
    c) obturator _____
    d) sciatic _____
    e) femoral _____

67. **Damage to the common peroneal nerve may result in**
    a) inability to dorsiflex the foot _____
    b) inability to plantar flex the foot _____
    c) anaesthesia on the dorsum of the foot except its borders _____
    d) anaesthesia on the sole of the foot _____
    e) anaesthesia on the medial border of foot _____

68. **The common peroneal nerve**
    a) ends by dividing into deep and superficial peroneal nerves _____
    b) may be injured lateral to the neck of the fibula _____
    c) forms a discrete component of the sciatic nerve _____
    d) arises from the dorsal divisions of the ventral rami of L4, L5, S1 and S2 _____
    e) if paralysed may result in inability to evert the foot _____

69. **Loss of sensation of the skin on the medial aspect of the leg may indicate injury to**
    a) spinal nerves L3 and L4 _____
    b) the common peroneal nerve _____
    c) the femoral nerve _____
    d) the deep peroneal nerve _____
    e) the sural nerve _____

The Nervous System

66. a) **TRUE**
    b) **FALSE** The tibial nerve lies more in the midline.
    c) **FALSE**
    d) **FALSE**
    e) **FALSE**

67. a) **TRUE** All the dorsiflexors are supplied by the deep peroneal branch of the common peroneal nerve.
    b) **FALSE** The plantar flexors are supplied by the tibial nerve.
    c) **TRUE** Due to loss of superficial and deep peroneal branches.
    d) **FALSE** The sole of the foot is supplied by the tibial nerve.
    e) **FALSE** This region is supplied by the saphenous nerve.

68. a) **TRUE**
    b) **TRUE**
    c) **TRUE**
    d) **TRUE**
    e) **TRUE** Peroneus longus and peroneus brevis, which evert the foot, are supplied by the superficial peroneal nerve.

69. a) **TRUE** Through the saphenous nerve.
    b) **FALSE**
    c) **TRUE** The saphenous nerve is a branch of the femoral nerve.
    d) **FALSE**
    e) **FALSE**

The Nervous System

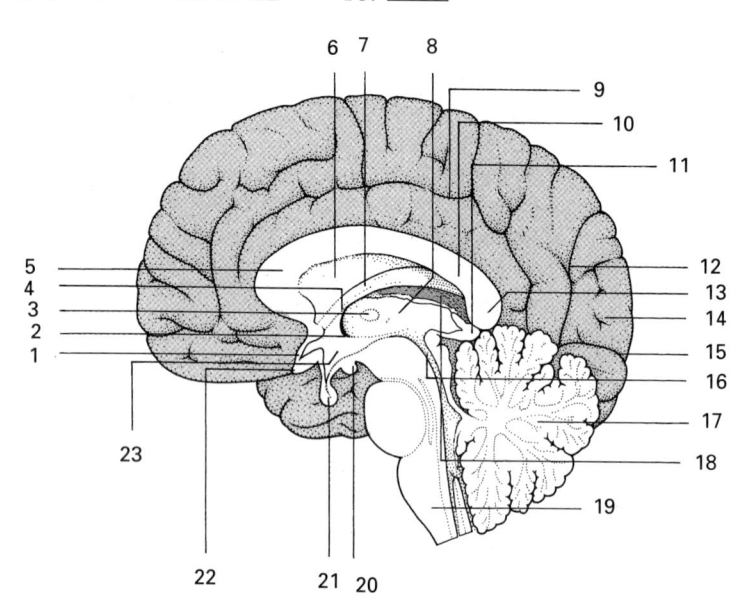

Picture questions

Identify the numbered structures in the following illustrations from the choices given

Question 1

1. _____
2. _____
3. _____
4. _____
5. _____
6. _____
7. _____
8. _____
9. _____
10. _____
11. _____
12. _____
13. _____
14. _____
15. _____
16. _____
17. _____
18. _____
19. _____
20. _____
21. _____
22. _____
23. _____

A. Genu of corpus callosum
B. Cerebral aqueduct
C. Hypothalamus
D. Cerebellum
E. Lamina terminalis
F. Septum pellucidum
G. Body of corpus callosum
H. Splenium of corpus callosum
I. Optic chiasma
J. Fornix
K. Thalamus
L. Hypothalamic sulcus
M. Cuneus
N. Parieto-occipital sulcus
O. Mamillary body
P. Medulla
Q. Thalamic interconnexus
R. Pituitary gland
S. Interventricular foramen
T. Cingulate sulcus
U. Posterior calcarine sulcus
V. Pineal gland
W. Choroid plexus

The Nervous System

Question 2
1. ___
2. ___
3. ___
4. ___
5. ___
6. ___
7. ___
8. ___
9. ___
10. ___
11. ___
12. ___
13. ___
14. ___
15. ___
16. ___
17. ___
18. ___
19. ___
20. ___
21. ___
22. ___
23. ___

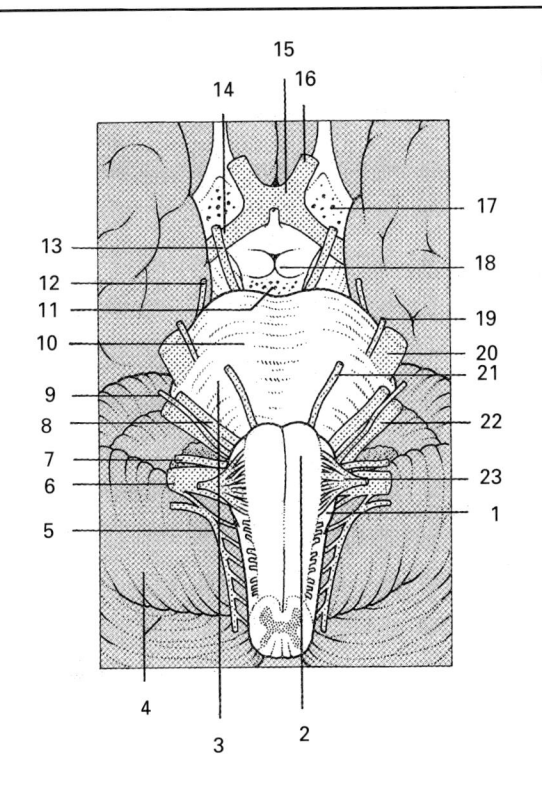

A. Trigeminal nerve (sensory root)
B. Nervus intermedius
C. Olive
D. Middle cerebellar peduncle
E. Optic chiasma
F. Pyramid
G. Hypoglossal nerve
H. Oculomotor nerve
I. Cerebellum
J. Abducens nerve
K. Glossopharyngeal nerve
L. Optic nerve
M. Posterior perforated substance
N. Optic tract
O. Accessory nerve
P. Vestibulocochlear nerve
Q. Mamillary body
R. Facial nerve
S. Trigeminal nerve (motor root)
T. Vagus nerve
U. Anterior perforated substance
V. Trochlear nerve
W. Pons

Answers on pages 152 and 153   135

The Nervous System

Question 3
1. ____
2. ____
3. ____
4. ____
5. ____
6. ____
7. ____
8. ____
9. ____

A. Ligamentum denticulatum
B. Dorsal root
C. Ventral root
D. Spinal nerve
E. Subarachnoid septum
F. Spinal pia mater
G. Arachnoid
H. Dura
I. Dorsal root ganglion

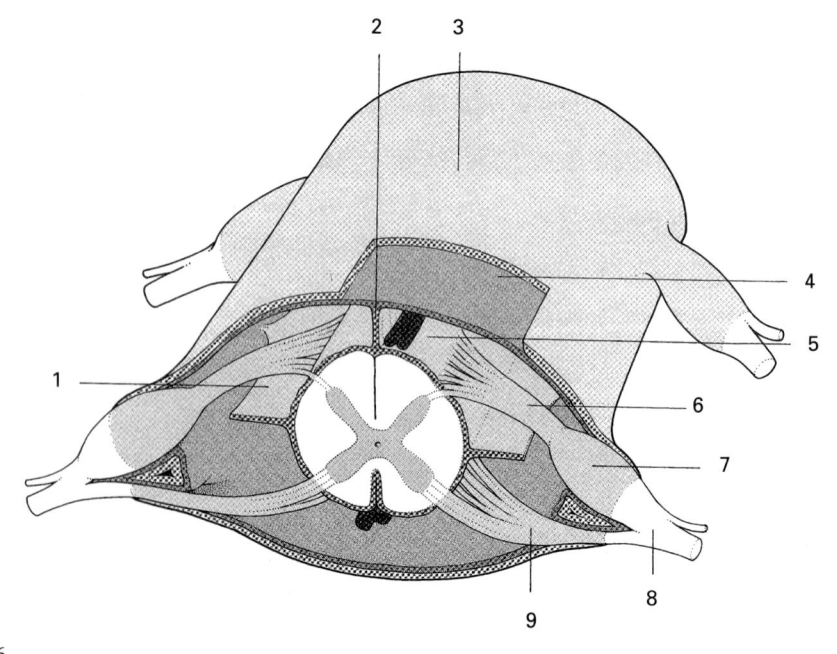

The Nervous System

Question 4
1. ____
2. ____
3. ____
4. ____
5. ____
6. ____
7. ____
8. ____
9. ____
10. ____
11. ____
12. ____
13. ____

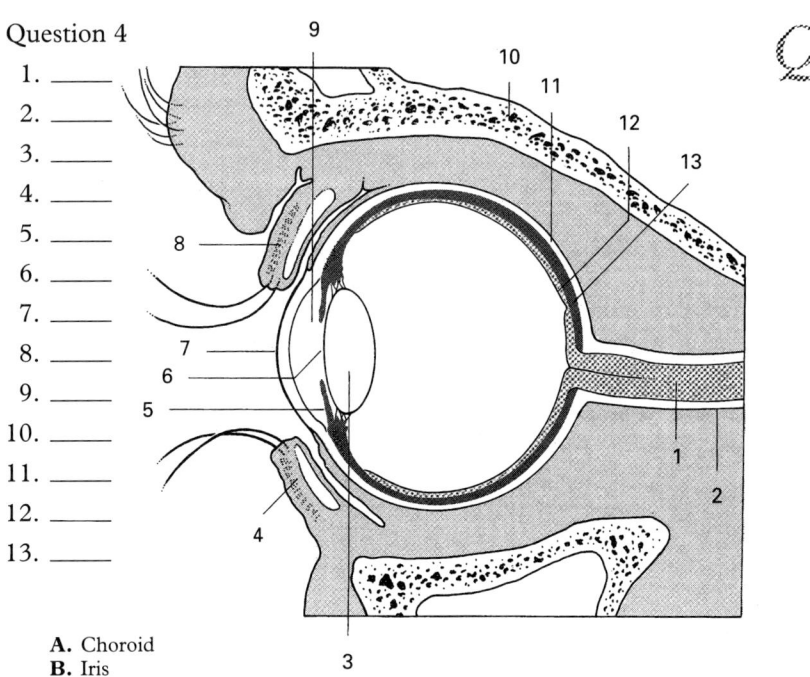

A. Choroid
B. Iris
C. Lens
D. Optic nerve
E. Upper eyelid
F. Wall of the orbit
G. Dura mater
H. Anterior chamber
I. Sclera
J. Retina
K. Lower eyelid
L. Cornea
M. Pupil

Answers on pages 153 and 154

The Nervous System

Question 5
1. ____
2. ____
3. ____
4. ____
5. ____
6. ____

A. Nasal cavity
B. Lacrimal sac
C. Lacrimal gland
D. Inferior lacrimal canaliculus
E. Nasolacrimal duct
F. Superior lacrimal canaliculus

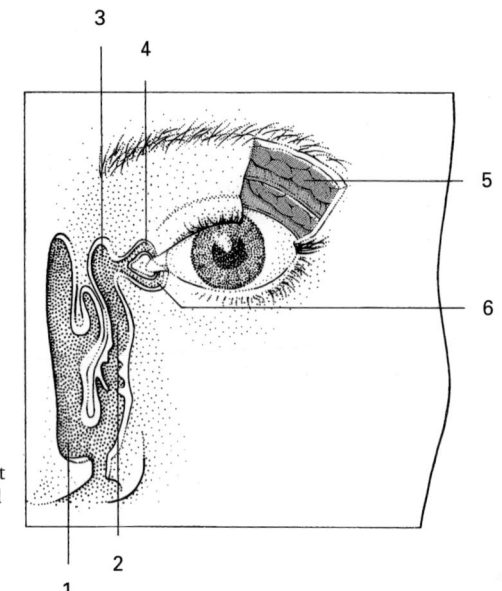

Question 6
1. ____
2. ____
3. ____
4. ____
5. ____
6. ____
7. ____
8. ____

A. Lateral geniculate body
B. Visual cortex
C. Optic tract
D. Medial half of retina
E. Optic nerve
F. Lateral half of retina
G. Optic chiasma
H. Optic radiation

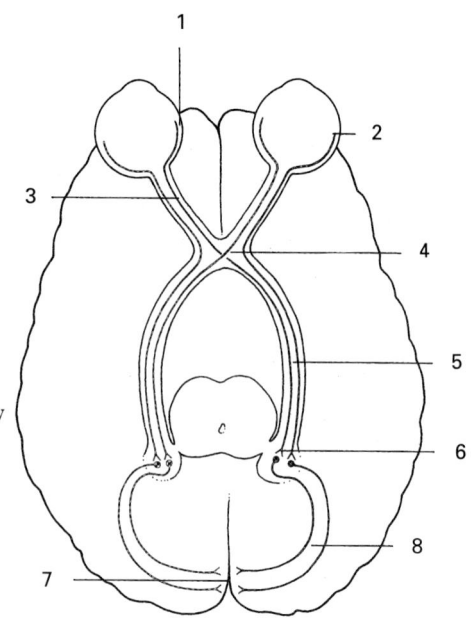

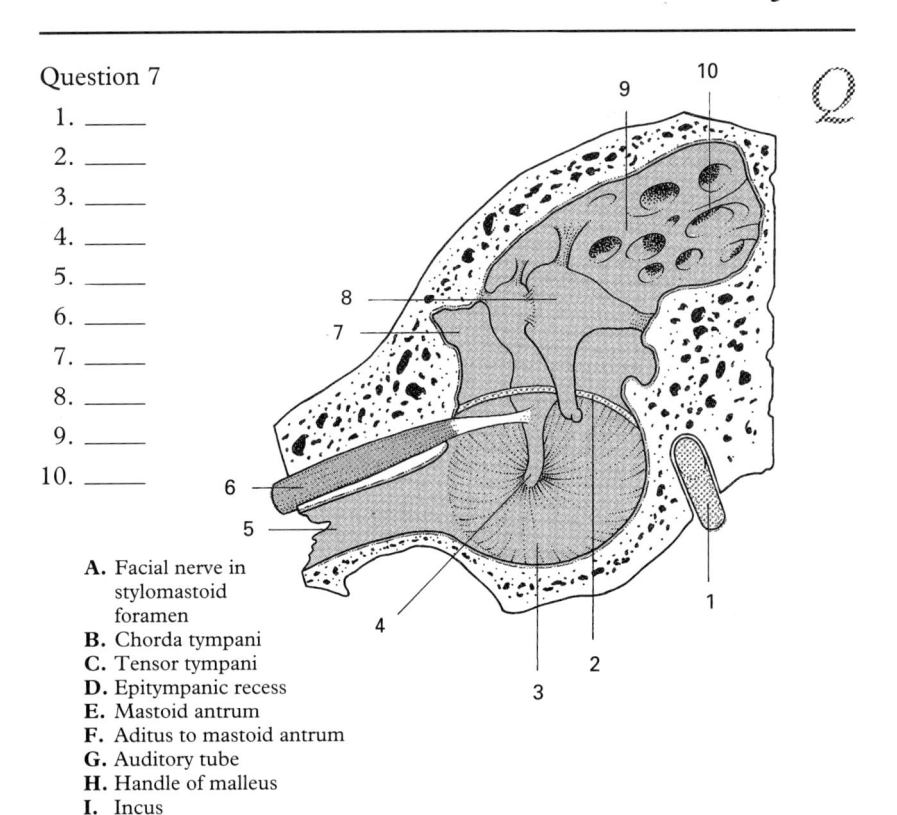

The Nervous System

Question 7
1. ____
2. ____
3. ____
4. ____
5. ____
6. ____
7. ____
8. ____
9. ____
10. ____

A. Facial nerve in stylomastoid foramen
B. Chorda tympani
C. Tensor tympani
D. Epitympanic recess
E. Mastoid antrum
F. Aditus to mastoid antrum
G. Auditory tube
H. Handle of malleus
I. Incus
J. Tympanic membrane

Answers on pages 154 and 155 139

The Nervous System

Question 8
1. ____
2. ____
3. ____
4. ____
5. ____
6. ____
7. ____
8. ____
9. ____
10. ____
11. ____
12. ____

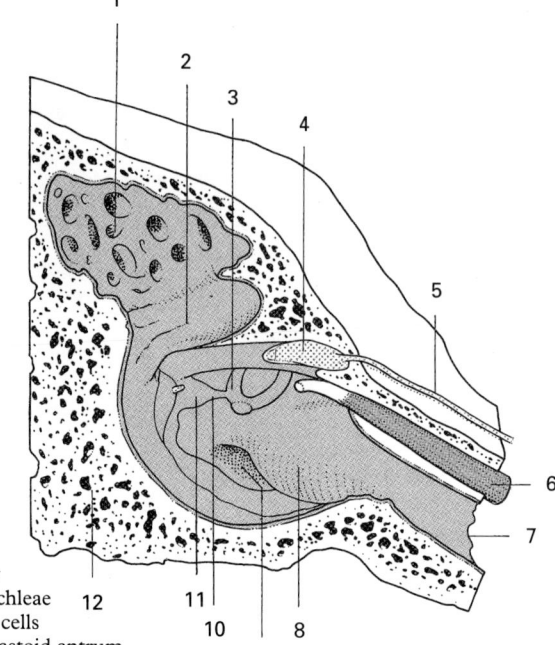

A. Promontory
B. Fenestra cochleae
C. Mastoid air cells
D. Aditus to mastoid antrum
E. Mastoid antrum
F. Tensor tympani
G. Greater petrosal nerve
H. Stapes
I. Facial nerve
J. Auditory tube
K. Pyramid
L. Tendon of stapedius

The Nervous System

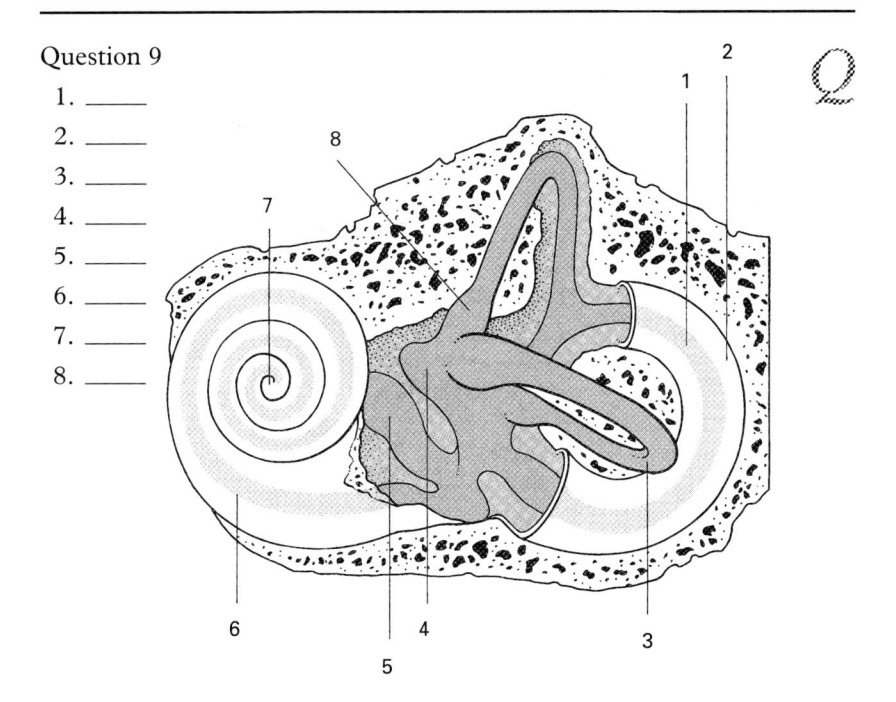

Question 9
1. ____
2. ____
3. ____
4. ____
5. ____
6. ____
7. ____
8. ____

A. Saccule
B. Posterior semicircular duct
C. Ampulla of anterior semicircular duct
D. Helicotrema
E. Posterior semicircular canal
F. Utricle
G. Lateral semicircular duct
H. Cochlear duct

Answers on page 155

The Nervous System

Question 12
1. ____
2. ____
3. ____
4. ____
5. ____
6. ____
7. ____
8. ____
9. ____
10. ____
11. ____

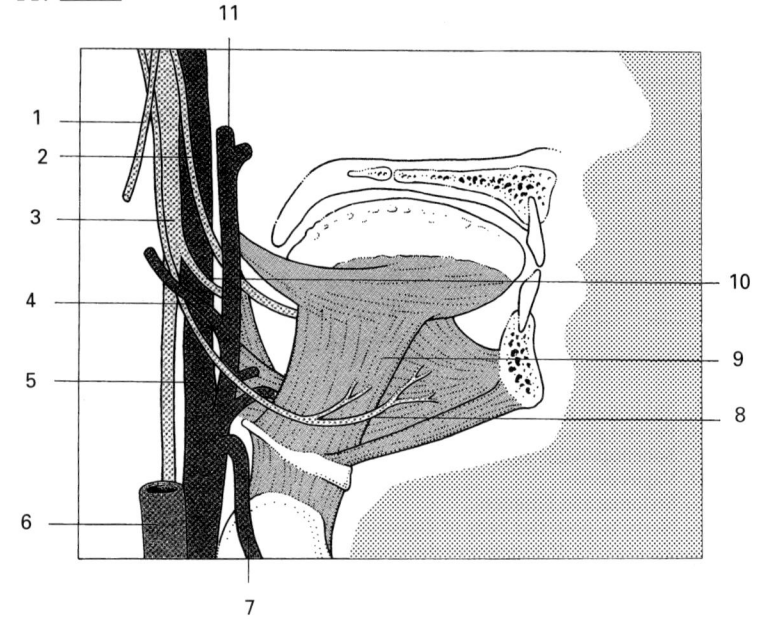

A. Glossopharyngeal nerve
B. Spinal accessory nerve
C. Occipital artery
D. External carotid artery
E. Pharyngeal branch of the vagus
F. Vagus nerve
G. Internal jugular vein
H. Internal carotid artery
I. Superior thyroid artery
J. Hyoglossus muscle
K. Hypoglossal nerve

The Nervous System

Question 13

1. ____
2. ____
3. ____
4. ____
5. ____
6. ____
7. ____
8. ____
9. ____
10. ____
11. ____
12. ____
13. ____
14. ____
15. ____
16. ____
17. ____
18. ____

19. ____
20. ____
21. ____
22. ____
23. ____
24. ____
25. ____
26. ____
27. ____
28. ____
29. ____
30. ____
31. ____
32. ____
33. ____
34. ____
35. ____
36. ____

A. C3
B. T12
C. S2
D. L4
E. S1
F. L1
G. T9
H. T2
I. C5
J. C7
K. C2
L. T2
M. S5
N. L2
O. L5
P. L5
Q. T4
R. C4

S. C8
T. C5
U. L1
V. L4
W. L2
X. C6
Y. T2
Z. C3
AA. C4
BB. S4
CC. L3
DD. T1
EE. T3
FF. L3
GG. S3
HH. S1
II. L5
JJ. S3

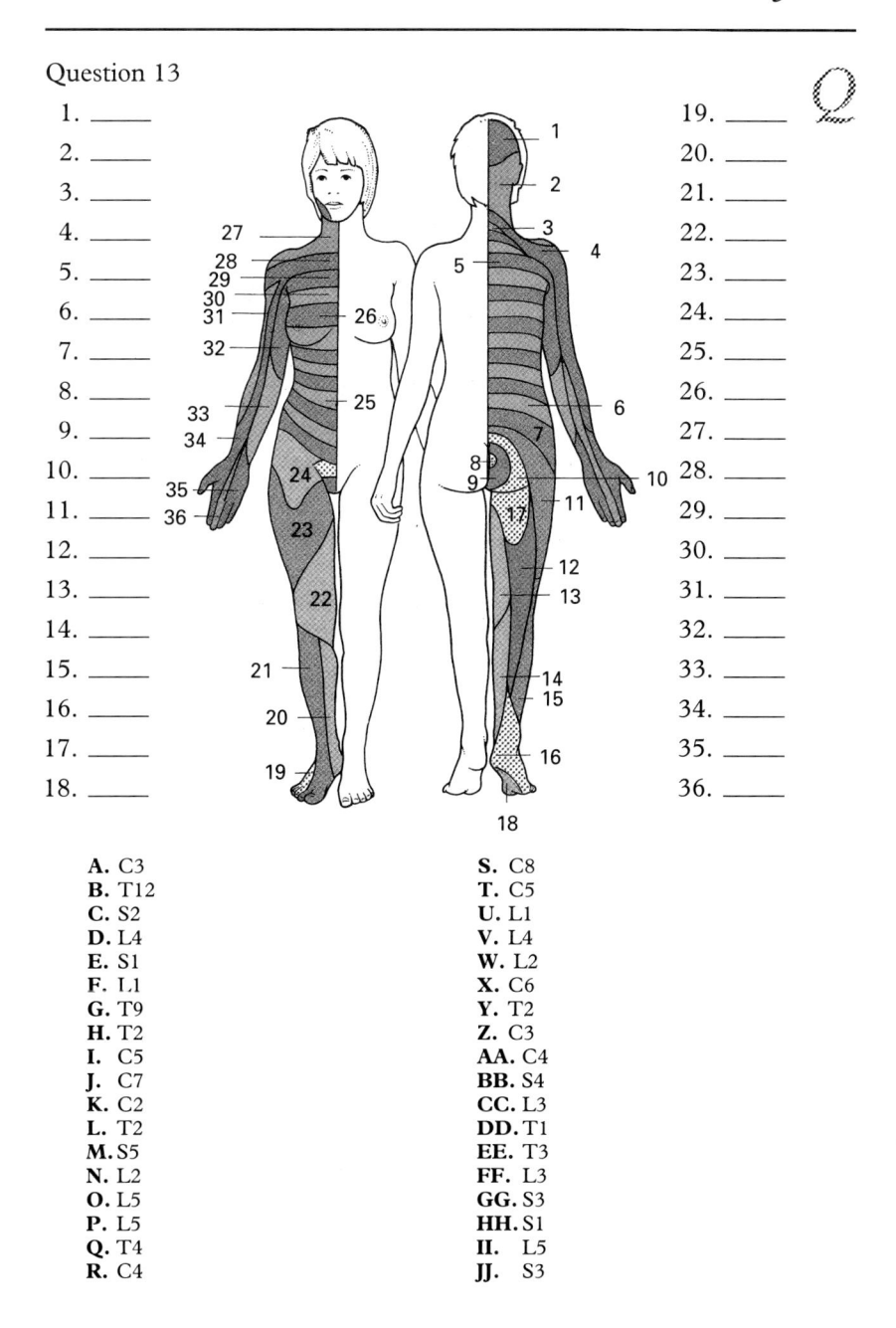

Answers on page 157

The Nervous System

Question 14

1. ____
2. ____
3. ____
4. ____
5. ____
6. ____
7. ____
8. ____
9. ____
10. ____
11. ____
12. ____
13. ____
14. ____
15. ____
16. ____
17. ____

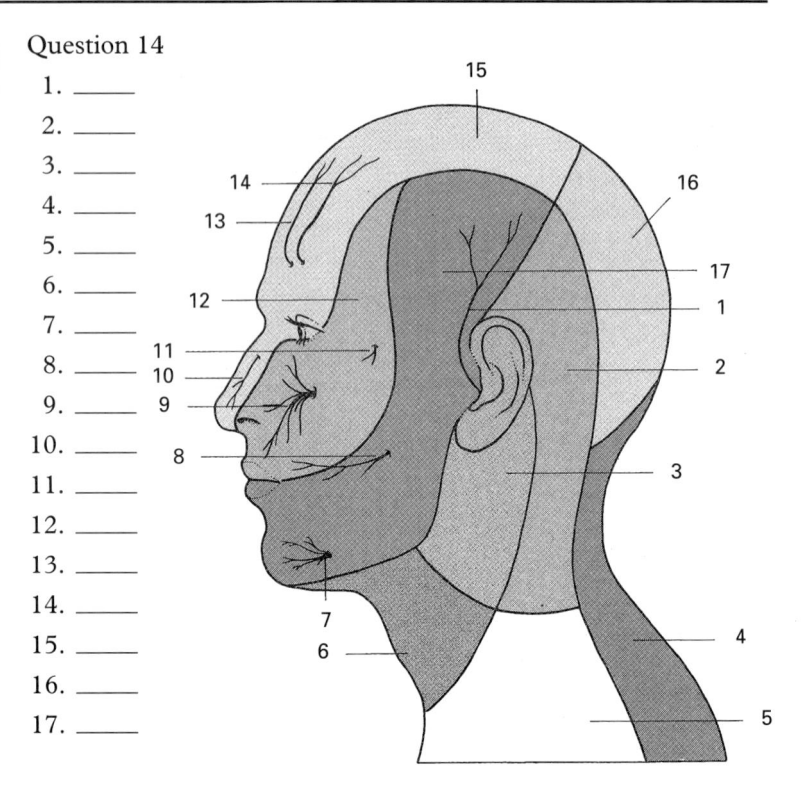

A. Ophthalmic nerve
B. Zygomaticofacial nerve
C. Dorsal rami of C3, C4, C5
D. Lesser occipital nerve (C2)
E. Mandibular nerve
F. Greater occipital nerve (C2, C3)
G. External nasal nerve
H. Supraclavicular nerves (C3, C4)
I. Transverse cervical nerve (C2, C3)
J. Infraorbital nerve
K. Auriculotemporal nerve
L. Mental nerve
M. Maxillary nerve
N. Supraorbital nerve
O. Buccal nerve
P. Supratrochlear nerve
Q. Greater auricular nerve

The Nervous System

Question 15
1. ____
2. ____
3. ____
4. ____
5. ____
6. ____
7. ____
8. ____
9. ____
10. ____
11. ____
12. ____
13. ____
14. ____

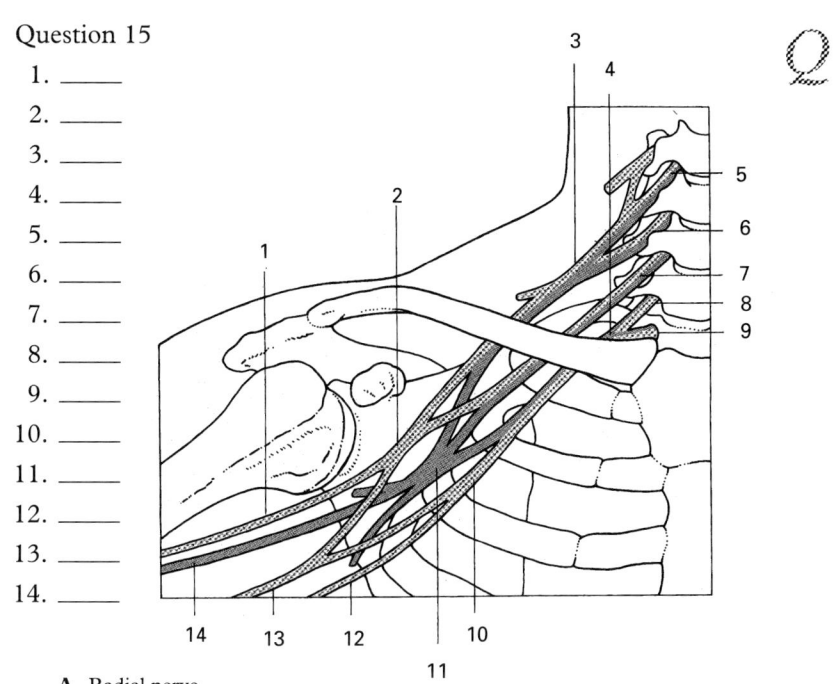

A. Radial nerve
B. Ulnar nerve
C. C7
D. Medial cord
E. Musculocutaneous nerve
F. C5
G. C8
H. Upper trunk
I. C6
J. Lateral cord
K. Lower trunk
L. T1
M. Median nerve
N. Posterior cord

Answers on page 158

The Nervous System

Question 16
1. ____
2. ____
3. ____
4. ____
5. ____
6. ____
7. ____
8. ____

A. Axillary nerve
B. Nerve to anconeus
C. Radial nerve
D. Deep terminal branch of radial nerve (posterior interosseus nerve)
E. Nerve to triceps
F. Supinator muscle
G. Lower lateral cutaneous nerve of arm
H. Superficial terminal branch of radial nerve

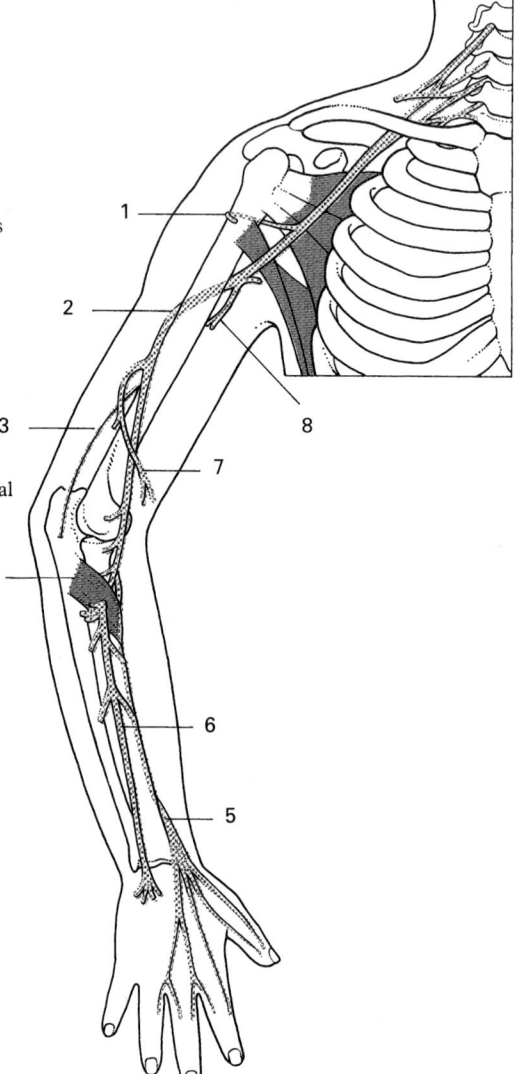

The Nervous System

Question 17

1. ____
2. ____
3. ____
4. ____
5. ____
6. ____
7. ____
8. ____
9. ____
10. ____
11. ____
12. ____
13. ____

A. Pontine arteries
B. Posterior cerebral artery
C. Anterior choroid artery
D. Anterior spinal artery
E. Posterior inferior cerebellar artery
F. Anterior cerebral artery
G. Middle cerebral artery
H. Vertebral artery
I. Superior cerebellar artery
J. Internal carotid artery
K. Anterior inferior cerebellar artery
L. Basilar artery
M. Posterior communicating artery

The Nervous System

Question 18
1. ____
2. ____
3. ____
4. ____
5. ____
6. ____
7. ____
8. ____
9. ____
10. ____

A. Tentorium cerebelli
B. Superior sagittal sinus
C. Cavernous sinus
D. Inferior petrosal sinus
E. Right transverse sinus
F. Sphenoparietal sinus
G. Straight sinus
H. Falx cerebri
I. Inferior sagittal sinus
J. Superior petrosal sinus

The Nervous System

Question 19
1. ___
2. ___
3. ___
4. ___
5. ___
6. ___
7. ___
8. ___
9. ___
10. ___
11. ___
12. ___
13. ___
14. ___

A. Diaphragma sellae
B. Cavernous sinus
C. Oculomotor nerve
D. Internal carotid artery
E. Trochlear nerve
F. Optic nerve
G. Hypophyseal stalk
H. Hypophysis cerebri
I. Arachnoid
J. Sphenoid air sinus
K. Pia mater
L. Ophthalmic nerve
M. Maxillary nerve
N. Abducens nerve

The Nervous System

A Picture questions

Question 1
1. **E** Lamina terminalis
2. **L** Hypothalamic sulcus
3. **Q** Thalamic interconnexus
4. **S** Interventricular foramen
5. **A** Genu of corpus callosum
6. **F** Septum pellucidum
7. **J** Fornix
8. **K** Thalamus
9. **T** Cingulate sulcus
10. **G** Body of corpus callosum
11. **V** Pineal gland
12. **N** Parieto-occipital sulcus
13. **H** Splenium of corpus callosum
14. **M** Cuneus
15. **U** Posterior calcarine sulcus
16. **B** Cerebral aqueduct
17. **D** Cerebellum
18. **W** Choroid plexus
19. **P** Medulla
20. **O** Mamillary body
21. **R** Pituitary gland
22. **I** Optic chiasma
23. **C** Hypothalamus

The Nervous System

Question 2
1. **C** Olive
2. **F** Pyramid
3. **D** Middle cerebellar peduncle
4. **I** Cerebellum
5. **O** Accessory nerve
6. **T** Vagus nerve
7. **K** Glossopharyngeal nerve
8. **R** Facial nerve
9. **B** Nervus intermedius
10. **W** Pons
11. **M** Posterior perforated substance
12. **V** Trochlear nerve
13. **H** Oculomotor nerve
14. **N** Optic tract
15. **E** Optic chiasma
16. **L** Optic nerve
17. **U** Anterior perforated substance
18. **Q** Mamillary body
19. **S** Trigeminal nerve (motor root)
20. **A** Trigeminal nerve (sensory root)
21. **J** Abducens nerve
22. **P** Vestibulocochlear nerve
23. **G** Hypoglossal nerve

Question 3
1. **A** Ligamentum denticulatum
2. **E** Subarachnoid septum
3. **H** Dura
4. **G** Arachnoid
5. **F** Spinal pia mater
6. **B** Dorsal root
7. **I** Dorsal root ganglion
8. **D** Spinal nerve
9. **C** Ventral root

The Nervous System

A Question 10
1. **E** Parotid gland
2. **I** Otic ganglion
3. **A** Mandibular nerve
4. **D** Ophthalmic nerve
5. **G** Maxillary nerve
6. **L** Frontal nerve
7. **O** Nasociliary nerve
8. **B** Ciliary ganglion
9. **P** Sphenopalatine ganglion
10. **N** Infraorbital nerve
11. **C** Lingual nerve
12. **H** Submandibular ganglion
13. **K** Inferior alveolar nerve
14. **M** Nerve to mylohyoid
15. **J** Nerve to tensor palati
16. **F** Tensor tympani muscle

Question 11
1. **D** Vagus nerve
2. **I** To muscles of facial expression
3. **B** Parotid gland
4. **K** Nerve to stylohyoid
5. **F** Nerve to posterior belly of digastric
6. **G** To muscles of auricle and occipitalis muscle
7. **E** Stylomastoid foramen
8. **L** Sensory fibres accompanying the auricular branch of vagus
9. **M** Internal acoustic meatus
10. **J** Geniculate ganglion
11. **N** Greater petrosal nerve
12. **C** Sphenopalatine ganglion
13. **S** Lacrimal gland
14. **P** Tongue
15. **A** Sublingual gland
16. **O** Submandibular gland
17. **R** Submandibular ganglion
18. **Q** Chorda tympani nerve
19. **H** Nerve to stapedius

The Nervous System

Question 12
1. **B** Spinal accessory nerve
2. **A** Glossopharyngeal nerve
3. **F** Vagus nerve
4. **C** Occipital artery
5. **H** Internal carotid artery
6. **G** Internal jugular vein
7. **I** Superior thyroid artery
8. **K** Hypoglossal nerve
9. **J** Hyoglossus muscle
10. **E** Pharyngeal branch of the vagus
11. **D** External carotid artery

Question 13
1. **K** C2
2. **A** C3
3. **AA** C4
4. **T** C5
5. **L** T2
6. **B** T12
7. **U** L1
8. **M** S5
9. **BB** S4
10. **GG** S3
11. **N** L2
12. **C** S2
13. **FF** L3
14. **D** L4
15. **O** L5
16. **HH** S1
17. **JJ** S3
18. **II** L5
19. **E** S1
20. **V** L4
21. **P** L5
22. **CC** L3
23. **W** L2
24. **F** L1
25. **G** T9
26. **Q** T4
27. **Z** C3
28. **R** C4
29. **H** T2
30. **EE** T3
31. **I** C5
32. **Y** T2
33. **DD** T1
34. **X** C6
35. **S** C8
36. **J** C7

The Nervous System

Question 14
1. **K** Auriculotemporal nerve
2. **D** Lesser occipital nerve (C2)
3. **Q** Greater auricular nerve
4. **C** Dorsal rami of C3, C4, C5
5. **H** Supraclavicular nerves (C3, C4)
6. **I** Transverse cervical nerve (C2, C3)
7. **L** Mental nerve
8. **O** Buccal nerve
9. **J** Infraorbital nerve
10. **G** External nasal nerve
11. **B** Zygomaticofacial nerve
12. **M** Maxillary nerve
13. **P** Supratrochlear nerve
14. **N** Supraorbital nerve
15. **A** Ophthalamic nerve
16. **F** Greater occipital nerve (C2, C3)
17. **E** Mandibular nerve

Question 15
1. **E** Musculocutaneous nerve
2. **J** Lateral cord
3. **H** Upper trunk
4. **K** Lower trunk
5. **F** C5
6. **I** C6
7. **C** C7
8. **G** C8
9. **L** T1
10. **D** Medial cord
11. **N** Posterior cord
12. **B** Ulnar nerve
13. **M** Median nerve
14. **A** Radial nerve

The Nervous System

Question 16
1. **A** Axillary nerve
2. **C** Radial nerve
3. **B** Nerve to anconeus
4. **F** Supinator muscle
5. **H** Superficial terminal branch of radial nerve
6. **D** Deep terminal branch of radial nerve (posterior interosseus nerve)
7. **G** Lower lateral cutaneous nerve of arm
8. **E** Nerve to triceps

Question 17
1. **F** Anterior cerebral artery
2. **J** Internal carotid artery
3. **M** Posterior communicating artery
4. **B** Posterior cerebral artery
5. **A** Pontine arteries
6. **K** Anterior inferior cerebellar artery
7. **E** Posterior inferior cerebellar artery
8. **D** Anterior spinal artery
9. **H** Vertebral artery
10. **L** Basilar artery
11. **I** Superior cerebellar artery
12. **C** Anterior choroid artery
13. **G** Middle cerebral artery

Question 18
1. **D** Inferior petrosal sinus
2. **A** Tentorium cerebelli
3. **G** Straight sinus
4. **E** Right transverse sinus
5. **H** Falx cerebri
6. **B** Superior sagittal sinus
7. **I** Inferior sagittal sinus
8. **J** Superior petrosal sinus
9. **F** Sphenoparietal sinus
10. **C** Cavernous sinus

The Nervous System

A Question 19
1. **C** Oculomotor nerve
2. **B** Cavernous sinus
3. **E** Trochlear nerve
4. **K** Pia mater
5. **L** Ophthalmic nerve
6. **I** Arachnoid
7. **M** Maxillary nerve
8. **N** Abducens nerve
9. **D** Internal carotid artery
10. **J** Sphenoid air sinus
11. **H** Hypophysis cerebri
12. **G** Hypophyseal stalk
13. **F** Optic nerve
14. **A** Diaphragma sellae

The Nervous System

Clinical problems

1. A patient referred to a neurologist was diagnosed as having a space-occupying intracranial lesion. She was complaining of severe headache, nausea and vomiting and on examination was found to have papilloedema — swelling of the optic disc. Why do space-occupying lesions such as intracranial tumours produce these changes? How does one examine the optic disc?

2. As a result of a blow on the head, a patient is suspected of having an extradural, subdural, or subarachnoid haemorrhage. What are the differences between these regarding their anatomical locations and the type of vessels ruptured?

3. A sample of CSF is usually obtained by doing a lumbar puncture. A trocar and cannula is inserted into the space between the spinous processes of the L3 and L4 vertebrae. On entering the subarachnoid space the cannula is withdrawn and clear CSF is seen dripping from the trocar. How does one identify the L3–L4 spinous processes? Why is this procedure done at this particular level? What structures do the trocar and cannula pass through before reaching the subarachnoid space?

The Nervous System

A Clinical problems

1. A space-occupying lesion will raise the intracranial pressure as there is no extra space within the rigid cranial cavity to accommodate the expanding mass. Headache is produced by compression of the dura. Pain fibres of the dura are distributed along its blood vessels. Nausea and vomiting may be due to compression of vomiting centres in the brainstem. Papilloedema is due to compression of the optic nerve. The subarachnoid space and the CSF extend all along the optic nerve and the increased pressure is transmitted onto the nerve. The optic disc is examined by ophthalmoscopy. The disc has a circular profile and is paler than the rest of the retina. It is medial to the macula, which has the centre for acute vision — the fovea centralis.

2. An extradural haemorrhage is usually due to rupture of middle meningeal vessels and is located between the meningeal layer of dura and the inner periosteum of bone. The meningeal vessels are periosteal vessels. A subdural haemorrhage occurs into the space between the dura and arachnoid and is usually due to rupture of cerebral veins. A subarachnoid haemorrhage is bleeding into the space between the arachnoid and the pia and can be due to rupture of cerebral vessels in the subarachnoid space.

3. The space between the L3 and L4 spines lies where a line joining the highest points of the iliac crest meets the midline. This is well below the lower end of the spinal cord (conus medullaris). In the adult, the cord ends at the lower border of the L1 vertebra. The subarachnoid space and the CSF extend as far as the lower border of S2. The trocar and cannula will pass through skin, subcutaneous tissue, supraspinous and interspinous ligaments or the ligamentum flavum, dura and arachnoid before entering the subarachnoid space.

The Nervous System

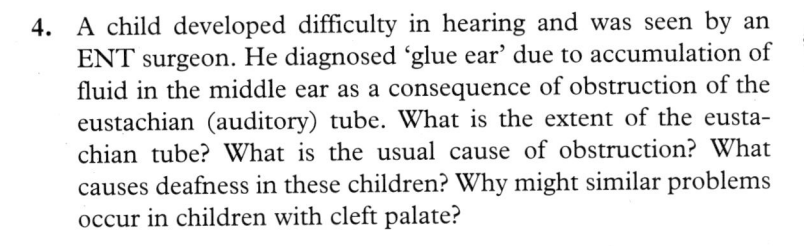

4. A child developed difficulty in hearing and was seen by an ENT surgeon. He diagnosed 'glue ear' due to accumulation of fluid in the middle ear as a consequence of obstruction of the eustachian (auditory) tube. What is the extent of the eustachian tube? What is the usual cause of obstruction? What causes deafness in these children? Why might similar problems occur in children with cleft palate?

5. A young man who fell on his outstretched hand and dislocated his shoulder has a suspected nerve injury as a complication of the shoulder dislocation. Which nerve is likely to be damaged in shoulder dislocations? How do you test for it? Which other injury in this region may damage the same nerve?

6. The median nerve may be compressed as it passes deep to the flexor retinaculum producing a condition known as the carpal tunnel syndrome. What is the carpal tunnel? What are the attachments of the flexor retinaculum? Which structures pass through the carpal tunnel? What would be the effect of compression of the median nerve in the carpal tunnel?

The Nervous System

4. The eustachian tube extends from the nasopharynx to the middle ear. It opens on the anterior wall of the middle ear and its patency is essential for the presence of air in the middle ear cavity. Obstruction is usually caused by throat infection and enlargement of the nasopharyngeal tonsil (adenoid) which lies very close to the opening of the tube in the pharynx. When the tube is obstructed, the air in the middle ear is replaced by fluid and this prevents vibration of the ossicles. Conduction deafness results. The tensor palatini and the levator palatini are the two muscles which normally open the eustachian tube. These do not function in children with cleft palate.

5. The axillary nerve is closely related to the inferior aspect of the shoulder joint. This supplies the deltoid and teres minor muscles and the skin over the upper lateral part of the arm. In a shoulder injury, damage to the nerve may be assessed by testing for cutaneous sensation over the insertion of deltoid. This area is not supplied by any other nerve. A fracture of the surgical neck of the humerus may also injure the axillary nerve.

6. The carpal tunnel is the space between the flexor retinaculum and the carpal bones. The flexor retinaculum is seen in the palm distal to the distal skin crease at the wrist and is attached to the pisiform and hook of the hamate medially, and the trapezium and the scaphoid laterally. Besides the median nerve, the carpal tunnel transmits the flexor digitorum superficialis and profundus tendons, and the tendons of flexor carpi radialis and flexor pollicis longus. All these tendons are covered by their respective synovial sheaths. Compression of the median nerve produces paraesthesia and other sensory changes over the palmar aspect of the lateral three digits. The skin on the palm of the hand will not be affected as it is supplied by the palmar branch of the median nerve which lies superficial to the retinaculum. The thenar muscles are supplied by the median nerve and these may be weak; but this effect is variable as these muscles are often also supplied by the ulnar nerve.

The Digestive System

The Digestive System

THE MOUTH AND PHARYNX

True/False

1. **With regard to the tongue:**
   a) the hypoglossal nerve supplies the extrinsic muscles
   b) the genioglossus pulls the tongue forward
   c) the chorda tympani nerve supplies the taste buds of the vallate papillae
   d) lymphatics from the whole of the side of the tongue drain into the submandibular lymph nodes
   e) the intrinsic muscles alter the shape of the tongue

2. **The following statements about the tongue are true:**
   a) the posterior third is developed from the third pharyngeal arch
   b) the muscles are developed from the occipital myotomes
   c) the lingual artery lies deep to the hyoglossus
   d) it has two lingual veins draining it on either side
   e) a lingual thyroid may occasionally be present at the foramen caecum

3. **The posterior third of tongue**
   a) is attached to the hyoid
   b) is covered by filiform papillae
   c) contains much lymphoid tissue
   d) has a nerve supply from the glossopharyngeal nerve
   e) is separated from the anterior two-thirds by the sulcus terminalis

The Digestive System

THE MOUTH AND PHARYNX

1. a) **TRUE** It supplies all the extrinsic and intrinsic muscles of the tongue except the palatoglossus.
   b) **TRUE** When one genioglossus is paralysed, the tongue deviates to the paralysed side when the patient is asked to protrude his tongue — a test for the hypoglossal nerve.
   c) **FALSE** The vallate papillae are supplied by the glossopharyngeal nerve. The taste buds in front of the vallate papillae are supplied by the chorda tympani nerve.
   d) **FALSE** The posterior third of the side of the tongue drains into the deep cervical nodes.
   e) **TRUE** And the extrinsic muscles move it in space.

2. a) **TRUE** The anterior two-thirds develop from the first arch.
   b) **TRUE** These myotomes are supplied by the hypoglossal nerve.
   c) **TRUE** And the lingual nerve lies superficial.
   d) **TRUE**
   e) **TRUE** The thyroglossal duct develops from the foramen caecum.

3. a) **TRUE** Through the hyoglossus muscle.
   b) **FALSE** All the papillae are in the anterior two-thirds.
   c) **TRUE** It has the lingual tonsil.
   d) **TRUE** The nerve also supplies the adjoining oropharynx.
   e) **TRUE** The sulcus terminalis is V-shaped, with the foramen caecum at its apex.

The Digestive System

4. **Regarding the teeth and gums:**
   a) the right central incisors are supplied by the right and left inferior alveolar nerves
   b) the inferior alveolar nerve supplies the lingual gingivae as well
   c) the labial gingivae of the upper teeth are supplied by the greater palatine nerves
   d) the deciduous teeth contain two premolars in each quadrant
   e) an infected tooth can sometimes produce earache

5. **The parotid gland**
   a) has a duct that pierces masseter to open into the vestibule of the mouth
   b) is mainly serous
   c) has the facial nerve passing through it deep to the external carotid artery
   d) is well encapsulated
   e) when acutely enlarged results in pain sensation being transmitted along the great auricular nerve

6. **The parotid gland**
   a) extends behind the temporomandibular joint
   b) is separated from the submandibular gland by the sphenomandibular ligament
   c) receives secretomotor fibres from the facial nerve
   d) receives secretomotor fibres which emerge from the brain in the glossopharyngeal nerve
   e) has a palpable duct

7. **The submandibular salivary gland is deep to**
   a) platysma
   b) deep fascia
   c) the facial artery
   d) the facial vein
   e) hyoglossus

The Digestive System

4. a) **TRUE** All the sensory nerves of each side in the mouth supply just beyond the midline.
   b) **FALSE** The inferior alveolar nerve supplies the outer gingiva on the lower jaw. The lingual gingiva is supplied by the lingual nerve.
   c) **FALSE** The labial gingivae are supplied by the superior alveolar nerves. The inner gingiva is supplied by the palatine nerves.
   d) **FALSE** Premolars are absent in the primary dentition.
   e) **TRUE** It is a referred pain through branches of the trigeminal nerve.

5. a) **FALSE** The duct lies on masseter and pierces buccinator opposite the second upper molar tooth to open into the vestibule.
   b) **TRUE**
   c) **FALSE** Structures in the gland from superficial to deep are the facial nerve, retromandibular vein and external carotid artery.
   d) **TRUE** The investing layer of the cervical fascia forms the capsule.
   e) **TRUE** Enlargement stretches the capsule, which is innervated by the great auricular nerve.

6. a) **TRUE** The superior surface is behind the temporomandibular joint and is also closely related to the external auditory meatus.
   b) **FALSE** It is the stylomandibular ligament that separates the two glands.
   c) **FALSE** The facial nerve at this level supplies the muscles of facial expression.
   d) **TRUE** These fibres synapse in the otic ganglion.
   e) **TRUE** The duct may be palpated on masseter on clenching the teeth.

7. a) **TRUE** Platysma is in the superficial fascia.
   b) **TRUE** The deep fascia splits to enclose the gland.
   c) **FALSE** The facial artery is embedded in the posterior aspect of the gland and partly lies deep to the gland.
   d) **TRUE** The vein crosses superficial to the gland.
   e) **FALSE** The gland is superficial to hyoglossus. The deep and superficial parts of the gland are separated by the mylohyoid muscle.

The Digestive System

8. **In operations on the submandibular gland the following are at risk:**
   a) cervical branch of the facial nerve
   b) hypoglossal nerve
   c) lingual nerve
   d) glossopharyngeal nerve
   e) mandibular branch of the facial nerve

9. **The soft palate**
   a) contains muscles supplied by the greater palatine nerve
   b) is covered on its undersurface by ciliated columnar epithelium
   c) contains a core of hyaline cartilage
   d) contains an aponeurosis derived from tensor palati
   e) rises to meet the posterior wall of the pharynx during swallowing

10. **The palatine tonsil is supplied by**
    a) the glossopharyngeal nerve
    b) the lesser palatine nerve
    c) the hypoglossal nerve
    d) the internal laryngeal nerve
    e) the pharyngeal branch of the vagus

11. **The palatine tonsil**
    a) is derived from the second pharyngeal arch
    b) is covered by columnar epithelium
    c) is supplied by the facial artery
    d) is related to the superior constrictor
    e) drains lymph to the jugulo-digastric lymph node

The Digestive System

8. a) **TRUE**   It crosses the superficial part of the gland posteriorly.
    b) **TRUE**   The hypoglossal nerve is related to the deep part of the gland deep to the mylohyoid muscle.
    c) **TRUE**   The lingual nerve is also related to the deep part of the gland.
    d) **FALSE** It lies deep to hyoglossus.
    e) **TRUE**   It often lies on the gland as it loops down below the mandible.

9. a) **FALSE** The greater palatine nerve gives sensory innervation to the mucosa of the hard palate.
    b) **FALSE** The undersurface is covered by the stratified squamous epithelium of the oral cavity. The nasal surface is lined by ciliated columnar epithelium.
    c) **FALSE** The soft palate is made of striated muscle.
    d) **TRUE**   This forms the core to which the other muscles are attached.
    e) **TRUE**   The palate is approximated against the palatopharyngeal sphincter (Passavant's ridge) on the superior constrictor.

10. a) **TRUE**   It is the nerve of the tonsillar fossa.
    b) **TRUE**   This also supplies the tonsillar bed.
    c) **FALSE** The hypoglossal is the motor nerve of the tongue.
    d) **FALSE** This is the sensory nerve of the laryngeal part of the pharynx and the upper part of the larynx.
    e) **FALSE** This is the motor nerve of the muscles of the pharynx and soft palate.

11. a) **FALSE** It is derived from the second pharyngeal pouch.
    b) **FALSE** It is covered by stratified squamous epithelium.
    c) **TRUE**   Also by branches from the ascending pharyngeal, ascending palatine and lingual arteries.
    d) **TRUE**   The palatine tonsil lies on the superior constrictor.
    e) **TRUE**   The node may be palpable behind the angle of the jaw in chronic tonsillitis.

The Digestive System

12. The piriform fossa

   a) is lined by ciliated epithelium   _____

   b) drains lymph to the deep cervical lymph nodes   _____

   c) has its mucous membrane supplied by the internal laryngeal nerve   _____

   d) is a usual site for lodging foreign bodies   _____

   e) can be clearly visualised in indirect laryngoscopy   _____

The Digestive System

12. a) **FALSE** It is lined by stratified squamous epithelium.
    b) **TRUE** Malignant tumours in the piriform fossa metastasise into these nodes.
    c) **TRUE** The trunk of the nerve lies just under the mucosa and can be anaesthetised by topical application of anaesthetic agents.
    d) **TRUE** Such as fish bones. Their removal may damage the internal laryngeal nerve.
    e) **FALSE** The piriform fossa is difficult to see and an early tumour in this area may be missed during indirect laryngoscopy.

The Digestive System

THE OESOPHAGUS AND STOMACH

True/False

13. The oesophagus
   a) is approximately 25 cm long in adults _____
   b) begins at the level of the cricoid cartilage _____
   c) has a mucous membrane containing a muscularis mucosa _____
   d) has a narrowing at the diaphragmatic hiatus _____
   e) is innervated by the recurrent laryngeal nerves _____

14. The oesophagus
   a) begins at the level of the sixth cervical vertebra _____
   b) is crossed anteriorly by the thoracic duct _____
   c) has venous drainage wholly into the azygos veins _____
   d) is lined by pseudostratified columnar epithelium _____
   e) is separated from the right atrium by the oblique sinus _____

15. In the neck, the oesophagus is related to
   a) the trachea anteriorly _____
   b) the recurrent laryngeal nerves _____
   c) the lateral lobes of the thyroid gland _____
   d) the subclavian artery _____
   e) the sympathetic trunk _____

16. The oesophagus in the mediastinum
   a) is related to the arch of the aorta _____
   b) is crossed anteriorly by the right bronchus _____
   c) is crossed anteriorly by the descending aorta _____
   d) has the recurrent laryngeal nerves lying in the groove between it and the trachea _____
   e) has a nerve plexus mostly contributed by the sympathetic trunk _____

The Digestive System

THE OESOPHAGUS AND STOMACH

13. a) **TRUE**
    b) **TRUE** The oesophagus is a continuation of the pharynx.
    c) **TRUE** The muscularis mucosa separates the mucosa from the submucosa and is continuous with that of the stomach.
    d) **TRUE** It passes through the diaphragm at the level of T10.
    e) **TRUE** Only the upper part is innervated by these nerves. The remainder receives direct branches from the vagus.

14. a) **TRUE** The cricoid cartilage lies at this level.
    b) **FALSE** It crosses behind the oesophagus from right to left.
    c) **FALSE** The lower end of the oesophagus is an important site of portosystemic anastomosis.
    d) **FALSE** The oesophagus is lined by stratified squamous epithelium throughout.
    e) **FALSE** It is separated from the left atrium by the oblique sinus of pericardium.

15. a) **TRUE** Throughout its course the trachea lies in front of the oesophagus.
    b) **TRUE** The recurrent laryngeal nerves lie in the groove between the trachea and the oesophagus.
    c) **TRUE** The lateral lobes, with the parathyroids, lie anterolateral to the oesophagus.
    d) **FALSE** The artery lies more laterally.
    e) **FALSE** The sympathetic trunk is also more lateral.

16. a) **TRUE** The arch of the aorta is related to the left side of the oesophagus.
    b) **FALSE** The left bronchus crosses it anteriorly, narrowing its lumen.
    c) **FALSE** The descending thoracic aorta crosses posterior to the oesophagus from left to right.
    d) **FALSE** Only the left recurrent laryngeal nerve is related to it in the mediastinum.
    e) **FALSE** The right and left vagus nerves supplying parasympathetic innervation predominate.

The Digestive System

Q

17. **At the upper end of the stomach**
    a) the cardiac orifice is at the level of the left ninth costal cartilage ____
    b) the fundus is at the level of the cardiac orifice ____
    c) a large bubble of air is always present in the fundus ____
    d) the left lobe of the liver is an anterior relation ____
    e) the cardiac sphincter is not visible but may be palpable ____

18. **At the pyloric region**
    a) the pyloric antrum is proximal to the pyloric canal ____
    b) the pyloric sphincter may be seen and felt at operation ____
    c) the pylorus is retroperitoneal ____
    d) the pylorus always lies at the transpyloric plane ____
    e) the prepyloric vein helps the surgeon to identify the pylorus ____

19. **The structures of the 'stomach bed' include**
    a) the body of the pancreas ____
    b) the spleen ____
    c) the right suprarenal gland ____
    d) the left suprarenal gland ____
    e) the transverse mesocolon ____

20. **The stomach has a blood supply from**
    a) the common hepatic artery ____
    b) the splenic artery ____
    c) the superior mesenteric artery ____
    d) the coeliac trunk ____
    e) the gastroduodenal artery ____

The Digestive System

17. a) **FALSE** The cardiac orifice lies at the level of the seventh costal cartilage.
   b) **FALSE** The fundus lies above the level of the cardiac orifice.
   c) **FALSE** A large bubble of air is present in the fundus in the erect posture.
   d) **TRUE**
   e) **FALSE** No anatomical sphincter exists at the cardiac end.

18. a) **TRUE**
   b) **TRUE** The sphincter consists of a thickening of circular muscle.
   c) **FALSE** The pylorus is completely invested by peritoneum.
   d) **FALSE** It is mobile and the position is variable.
   e) **TRUE** The vein crosses in front of the pylorus.

19. a) **TRUE** The pancreas lies behind the stomach, separated from it by the lesser sac.
   b) **TRUE**
   c) **FALSE**
   d) **TRUE** The left kidney also lies behind the stomach.
   e) **TRUE** The transverse mesocolon is attached to the anterior surface of the pancreas.

20. a) **TRUE** The common hepatic artery gives off the right gastric and the gastroduodenal arteries.
   b) **TRUE** The short gastric and left gastroepiploic arteries are branches of the splenic artery.
   c) **FALSE**
   d) **TRUE** The coeliac trunk gives off the left gastric, common hepatic and splenic arteries.
   e) **TRUE** The gastroduodenal artery supplies the greater curvature through the right gastroepiploic artery.

The Digestive System

21. **The lesser curvature of the stomach can be devascularised by ligating**
    a) the short gastric arteries
    b) the left gastric artery
    c) the splenic artery
    d) the left gastroepiploic artery
    e) the right gastric artery

22. **Regarding the peritoneal relations of the stomach:**
    a) the greater sac separates the anterior surface from the anterior abdominal wall
    b) the lesser sac separates the posterior surface from the posterior abdominal wall
    c) the free border of the lesser omentum is attached to the pylorus
    d) the greater omentum continues as the gastrosplenic ligament
    e) the greater omentum lies in front of the transverse colon

The Digestive System

21. a) **FALSE** The short gastric arteries supply the greater curvature of the stomach.
   b) **TRUE** The left and right gastric arteries anastomose along the lesser curvature.
   c) **FALSE** The splenic artery supplies the greater curvature.
   d) **FALSE** The left and right gastroepiploic arteries anastomose along the greater curvature.
   e) **TRUE**

22. a) **TRUE**
   b) **TRUE**
   c) **FALSE** It is attached to the duodenum about 1 inch from the pylorus.
   d) **TRUE** The greater omentum is attached to the greater curvature and merges with the gastrosplenic ligament on the left side.
   e) **TRUE** The greater omentum lies in front of the transverse colon and folds back on itself to attach to the transverse colon.

The Digestive System

THE PANCREAS AND INTESTINES

True/False

23. The following statements about the pancreas are true:
   a) the head is related to the duodenum
   b) the superior mesenteric vessels lie behind the uncinate process
   c) the portal vein is formed behind the neck
   d) the bile duct lies in front of the neck
   e) a tumour in the head may produce jaundice

24. The pancreas
   a) develops at the junction of midgut and hindgut
   b) has venous drainage mostly to the superior mesenteric vein
   c) has a blood supply from the inferior mesenteric artery
   d) has its main duct opening above the accessory duct
   e) has the splenic artery along its upper border

25. The tail of the pancreas
   a) lies in the gastrosplenic ligament
   b) is accompanied by the splenic artery
   c) is related to the spleen
   d) has numerous islets
   e) is ductless

The Digestive System

THE PANCREAS AND INTESTINES

23. a) **TRUE** The head lies in the concavity formed by the first, second and third parts of the duodenum.
    b) **FALSE** The vessels lie anterior to the uncinate process.
    c) **TRUE** The superior mesenteric and splenic veins join to form the portal vein.
    d) **FALSE** The bile duct lies in a groove on the posterior surface of the head of the pancreas before entering the duodenum.
    e) **TRUE** A tumour may compress the bile duct and produce obstructive jaundice.

24. a) **FALSE** The pancreas develops at the junction of foregut and midgut.
    b) **FALSE** The venous drainage is mostly to the splenic vein.
    c) **FALSE** The blood supply is from the splenic, superior mesenteric and gastroduodenal arteries.
    d) **FALSE** The accessory duct crosses the main duct and opens at a higher level.
    e) **TRUE** The splenic vein is closely applied to its posterior surface.

25. a) **FALSE** It is in the lienorenal ligament.
    b) **TRUE** The splenic artery enters the lienorenal ligament.
    c) **TRUE** The tail touches the spleen.
    d) **TRUE** More in the tail than elsewhere.
    e) **FALSE** The duct system is arranged in a herring-bone pattern and is present in all parts of the pancreas.

The Digestive System

26. **The pancreas**
    a) has two duct systems, developmentally
    b) has an accessory duct derived from part of the ventral pancreatic duct
    c) crosses behind the aorta and inferior vena cava
    d) receives vessels only from the coeliac trunk
    e) is retroperitoneal throughout

27. **The duodenum**
    a) is retroperitoneal throughout
    b) develops from the foregut and midgut
    c) is supplied entirely by branches of the coeliac trunk
    d) has no villi in the mucosa
    e) has Brunner's glands in the submucosa

28. **Concerning the first part of the duodenum:**
    a) it has the portal vein and bile duct posteriorly
    b) the gastroduodenal artery lies anteriorly
    c) the duodenal 'cap' is a radiographic feature
    d) the proximal part is mobile
    e) it is related to the gallbladder anteriorly

The Digestive System

26. a) **TRUE**   The pancreas develops from the ventral and dorsal pancreatic buds.
   b) **FALSE**   The accessory duct is derived from the terminal part of the dorsal pancreatic duct. The ventral pancreatic duct forms the terminal part of the main pancreatic duct.
   c) **FALSE**   The pancreas crosses anterior to the aorta and the inferior vena cava, and also the left kidney and the left suprarenal gland.
   d) **FALSE**   The inferior pancreaticoduodenal artery from the superior mesenteric artery supplies the head of the pancreas.
   e) **FALSE**   Most of the pancreas is retroperitoneal. The tail is in the lienorenal ligament.

27. a) **FALSE**   The first inch is completely covered by peritoneum.
   b) **TRUE**   The first part and half of the second part develop from the foregut, the rest from the midgut.
   c) **FALSE**   The inferior pancreaticoduodenal artery is a branch of the superior mesenteric artery.
   d) **FALSE**   The villi are present in all parts of the small intestine.
   e) **TRUE**   Their ducts open at the bases of the villi.

28. a) **TRUE**   Both structures continue up in the free edge of the lesser omentum.
   b) **FALSE**   The gastroduodenal artery, a branch of the common hepatic artery, lies posteriorly. Bleeding from this vessel is a complication of a duodenal ulcer on the posterior wall.
   c) **TRUE**   The first inch of the duodenum contributes to the triangular 'duodenal cap'.
   d) **TRUE**   It has a complete investment of peritoneum.
   e) **TRUE**   The body and neck of the gallbladder are directly related to the first part of the duodenum.

The Digestive System

29. **The second part of the duodenum**
   a) lies behind the hilum of the right kidney
   b) lies behind the gallbladder
   c) is crossed in front by the transverse mesocolon
   d) extends down to the lower border of L3 vertebra
   e) is supplied by the pancreaticoduodenal arteries

30. **The small intestine**
   a) has more lymphoid tissue in the proximal part
   b) has villi covered by columnar epithelium
   c) has more arterial arcades in the jejunal mesentery
   d) has more circular folds in the distal part
   e) is supplied entirely by the superior mesenteric artery

31. **A Meckel's diverticulum (ileal diverticulum)**
   a) is present in 22% of the population
   b) represents the remains of the urachus
   c) is usually situated at the junction between the jejunum and the ileum
   d) may contain gastric mucosa
   e) may be attached to the anterior abdominal wall

32. **With regard to the appendix:**
   a) it contains no lymphoid tissue
   b) the position of the base is inconstant
   c) it is supplied by a branch from the superior mesenteric artery
   d) the tip lies most commonly in the retrocaecal position
   e) it opens into the first 2.5 cm of the ascending colon

The Digestive System

29. a) **FALSE** It lies anterior to the hilum of the right kidney.
    b) **TRUE** The fundus of the gallbladder is related to the second part of the duodenum.
    c) **TRUE** The root of the transverse mesocolon is attached to the second part of the duodenum.
    d) **TRUE** The second part lies to the right of the L2 vertebra and extends down to L3.
    e) **TRUE** The superior and inferior pancreaticoduodenal arteries form an anastomosis along the duodenum.

30. a) **FALSE** The Peyer's patches are in the ileal mucosa.
    b) **TRUE** The villi are covered by a simple columnar epithelium.
    c) **FALSE** The ileal arcades are more numerous, with the terminal arteries short and straight.
    d) **FALSE** The jejunum contains more plicae circulares than does the ileum.
    e) **TRUE** The superior mesenteric artery supplies the entire midgut.

31. a) **FALSE** Only about 2% of the population have an ileal diverticulum.
    b) **FALSE** A Meckel's diverticulum is a remnant of the vitelline duct.
    c) **FALSE** It is usually found about 2 feet from the ileocaecal valve.
    d) **TRUE** However, it normally contains ileal mucosa.
    e) **TRUE** It may be joined to the umbilicus by a fibrous cord.

32. a) **FALSE** There is a large amount of lymphoid tissue in the appendix.
    b) **FALSE** The base has a constant position and is on the posteromedial wall of the caecum below the ileocaecal opening.
    c) **TRUE** It is supplied by a branch of the posterior caecal artery.
    d) **TRUE** Such a position is due to the descent of the caecum and ascending colon during development.
    e) **FALSE** The appendix opens into the caecum.

The Digestive System

33. The caecum
   a) lies in the right iliac fossa
   b) is always retroperitoneal
   c) is normally palpable
   d) is related to the right psoas major muscle
   e) has the ileocaecal valve on the anterior wall

34. A loop of transverse colon can be identified because
   a) it has appendices epiploicae attached to it
   b) it has no circular folds
   c) it has longitudinal bands of muscles running along it
   d) it has no mesocolon
   e) it has no haustrations

35. The rectum
   a) is directly related posteriorly to the uterine cervix in the female
   b) has the sacral plexus behind it
   c) has a complete mesentery
   d) has taeniae coli continued onto it
   e) is supplied by the inferior rectal artery

36. With regard to the rectum:
   a) Waldeyer's fascia lies in front of it
   b) the middle rectal artery supplies the mucosa
   c) lymph drains partly into the inguinal nodes
   d) it has a dilated portion — the ampulla — in the upper part
   e) it is developed from the midgut and hindgut

The Digestive System

33. a) **TRUE**
    b) **FALSE** A retrocaecal fossa may be present, giving the caecum an almost complete peritoneal covering.
    c) **FALSE** A normal caecum is not palpable.
    d) **TRUE** It also rests on the right iliacus muscle.
    e) **FALSE** The valve is at the ileocaecal opening on the posteromedial wall.

34. a) **TRUE** They are present throughout the large intestine. The rectum does not have them.
    b) **TRUE** Circular folds (plicae circulares) are only present in the small intestine.
    c) **TRUE** The three bands — taeniae coli — extend along the length of the large intestine.
    d) **FALSE** The transverse colon and sigmoid colon have a mesocolon.
    e) **FALSE** These are present throughout the large intestine. The rectum has no haustrations.

35. a) **FALSE** The rectum lies behind the uterus and vagina separated by the rectouterine pouch.
    b) **TRUE** Posteriorly it is also related to the piriformis, coccygeus and levator ani muscles.
    c) **FALSE** The upper third is covered anteriorly and laterally by peritoneum, the middle third is covered anteriorly only, and the lower third of the rectum is devoid of peritoneum.
    d) **FALSE** The longitudinal muscle forms a complete investment externally.
    e) **FALSE** The inferior rectal artery supplies the anal canal.

36. a) **FALSE** Waldeyer's fascia is the condensation of pelvic fascia anchoring the rectum to the sacrum.
    b) **FALSE** The artery is small and it supplies the muscle.
    c) **FALSE** Lymph drains into the pararectal nodes and from there into the nodes accompanying the arteries supplying the rectum.
    d) **FALSE** The ampulla is in the lower part of the rectum, just above the pelvic floor.
    e) **FALSE** The rectum develops solely from the hindgut.

The Digestive System

37. **The anal canal**
    a) is a boundary of the ischiorectal fossa
    b) is surrounded by an involuntary external sphincter
    c) has an important angle to the rectum maintained by the puborectalis muscle
    d) drains its lymph to the common iliac nodes only
    e) is insensitive to pain

38. **With regard to the anal canal:**
    a) it lies behind the perineal body
    b) it is partly developed from ectoderm
    c) its longitudinal muscle coat forms the internal sphincter
    d) the anal columns are above the pectinate line
    e) it is lined throughout by columnar epithelium

39. **Structures normally felt on rectal examination are**
    a) the ureter
    b) the prostate
    c) the seminal vesicles
    d) the uterine cervix
    e) the rectovesical pouch

The Digestive System

37. a) **TRUE** The ischiorectal fossa is filled with fat, allowing the anal canal to expand into it during defaecation.
    b) **FALSE** The external sphincter is a striated muscle and is under voluntary control.
    c) **TRUE** The angle is maintained by the anorectal ring, formed by the fusion of the puborectalis sling and the deep part of the external sphincter.
    d) **FALSE** Lymph drains also into the inferior mesenteric and superficial inguinal nodes.
    e) **FALSE** The lower part of the anal canal has a somatic nerve supply.

38. a) **TRUE** The anal canal is separated from the bulb of the penis in the male and from the vagina in the female by the perineal body.
    b) **TRUE** The mucous membrane of the lower half is derived from ectoderm.
    c) **FALSE** The circular muscle forms the internal sphincter.
    d) **TRUE** The lower ends of the anal columns are joined together by the anal valves at the pectinate line.
    e) **FALSE** The lower half is lined by stratified squamous epithelium.

39. a) **FALSE**
    b) **TRUE**
    c) **FALSE** The seminal vesicles are palpable only if inflamed.
    d) **TRUE** It is palpable through the vaginal wall.
    e) **FALSE** Unless it contains malignant deposits.

The Digestive System

THE LIVER AND GALLBLADDER

True/False

40. **The line dividing the two functional lobes of the liver, across which the ducts, hepatic arteries and portal vein tributaries of each lobe do not pass, is one joining**
    a) the falciform ligament to the ligamentum venosum
    b) the quadrate lobe to the caudate lobe
    c) the gallbladder fossa to the ligamentum venosum
    d) the falciform ligament to the lesser omentum
    e) the gallbladder fossa to the inferior vena cava

41. **The common bile duct**
    a) is formed by the union of the right and left hepatic ducts
    b) enters the middle of the second part of the duodenum
    c) is accompanied by the common hepatic artery on its right side
    d) passes in front of the first part of the duodenum
    e) has no muscle tissue in its wall

42. **Concerning the liver:**
    a) it develops from the midgut
    b) it is related to the left suprarenal gland
    c) sinusoids drain to a central vein
    d) a prolongation of the lesser sac is related to the caudate lobe
    e) the fissure for the ligamentum venosum is a site of attachment of the lesser omentum

43. **With regard to the liver:**
    a) the sinusoids are also called spaces of Disse
    b) the portal vein is connected to the umbilical vein in the fetus
    c) two hepatic veins are seen at the porta hepatis
    d) hepatic cells are derived from the midgut
    e) it develops in the ventral mesogastrium

The Digestive System

THE LIVER AND GALLBLADDER

40. a) **FALSE** The falciform ligament is between the two anatomical lobes.
    b) **FALSE** The quadrate and caudate lobes are functionally part of the left lobe.
    c) **FALSE** The groove for the ligamentum venosum lies between the two anatomical lobes.
    d) **FALSE** The lesser omentum is attached to the groove for the ligamentum venosum.
    e) **TRUE**

41. a) **FALSE** The common bile duct is formed by the union of the cystic and common hepatic ducts.
    b) **TRUE** It pierces the duodenal wall with the main pancreatic duct.
    c) **FALSE** The common hepatic artery lies to the left of the bile duct.
    d) **FALSE** The bile duct passes behind the first part of the duodenum.
    e) **FALSE** There is an incomplete layer of smooth muscle in the wall of the bile duct.

42. a) **FALSE** The liver develops from the foregut into the septum transversum.
    b) **FALSE** The visceral surface is related to the right suprarenal gland.
    c) **TRUE** A single central vein lies within each lobule of the liver.
    d) **TRUE** The lesser sac ascends behind the caudate lobe.
    e) **TRUE**

43. a) **FALSE** The space of Disse separates the sinusoids from the hepatic cells.
    b) **TRUE** In the fetus the left umbilical vein (ligamentum teres in the adult) joins the left branch of the portal vein.
    c) **FALSE** The porta hepatis contains the portal vein. The hepatic veins are at the posterior surface.
    d) **FALSE** Hepatic cells are formed from the hepatic diverticulum which is an outgrowth of the foregut.
    e) **TRUE** The hepatic diverticulum grows into the ventral mesogastrium.

The Digestive System

44. The bare area of the liver
   a) is on the right lobe
   b) is related to the inferior vena cava
   c) is bounded by the two layers of the coronary ligament
   d) has a poor blood supply
   e) is a site of portosystemic anastomosis

45. The liver
   a) is completely surrounded by peritoneum
   b) is normally palpable in infants
   c) derives its blood supply from the superior mesenteric artery
   d) has the falciform ligament attached to the fissure for the ligamentum teres
   e) has sinusoids containing mixed arterial and venous blood

46. With regard to the liver:
   a) its cells are arranged in sheets
   b) its bile canaliculi are intercellular
   c) its blood supply mostly through the hepatic artery
   d) its lymph drains via the bile duct
   e) its lobules are bounded by portal triads

47. Regarding the relations of the liver:
   a) the oesophagus lies behind the caudate lobe
   b) the left kidney is a direct relation of the left lobe
   c) the right colic flexure is related to the right lobe
   d) the right suprarenal gland is related to the bare area
   e) the diaphragm separates the right surface from the right lung and pleura

The Digestive System

44. a) **TRUE** The bare area is on the diaphragmatic surface of the right lobe.
    b) **TRUE**
    c) **TRUE** The bare area is formed by the gap between the two layers of the coronary ligament.
    d) **FALSE** Its blood supply is similar to that of the rest of the liver.
    e) **TRUE** Small veins from the liver (portal vein) anastomose with veins draining the diaphragm (systemic veins).

45. a) **FALSE** The bare area on the posterior surface of the right lobe has no peritoneum.
    b) **TRUE** It is relatively larger in infants than in adults.
    c) **FALSE** The liver is supplied by the portal vein and the hepatic artery, usually a branch of the coeliac trunk. Occasionally the hepatic artery may arise from the superior mesenteric artery.
    d) **FALSE** It is attached to the anterior and superior surfaces of the liver and to the notch for the ligamentum teres on the inferior border.
    e) **TRUE** The branches of both the portal vein and the hepatic artery empty into the sinusoids.

46. a) **TRUE** Sheets of hepatic cells radiate from the central vein to the periphery of the lobule.
    b) **TRUE** They lie between hepatocytes.
    c) **FALSE** Only 20% of the blood supply is from the hepatic artery, the rest is from the portal vein.
    d) **FALSE** The liver has lymph vessels and through them lymph from the liver drains into the hepatic nodes at the porta hepatis.
    e) **TRUE** The portal triads consist of branches of the hepatic artery, portal vein and bile duct.

47. a) **FALSE** The oesophagus lies behind the left lobe of the liver.
    b) **FALSE** The right kidney is related to the inferior surface of the right lobe of the liver.
    c) **TRUE** The right colic (hepatic) flexure is related to the inferior surface of the right lobe.
    d) **TRUE**
    e) **TRUE**

The Digestive System

48. The gallbladder
   a) has a capacity of about 100 ml
   b) concentrates bile 5–10 times
   c) is related to the fourth part of the duodenum
   d) is usually supplied by a branch of the hepatic artery
   e) is palpable at the tip of the seventh costal cartilage

49. With regard to the gallbladder:
   a) it has smooth muscle in its wall
   b) the main stimulus for contraction is through the vagus nerve
   c) its blood supply is entirely from the cystic artery
   d) filling is regulated by valves in the neck
   e) contraction is stimulated by cholecystokinin

The Digestive System

48. a) **FALSE**   It has a capacity of 50–70 ml.
    b) **TRUE**   It concentrates the bile up to 12-fold.
    c) **FALSE**   It is related to the first and second parts of the duodenum.
    d) **TRUE**   The cystic artery.
    e) **FALSE**   Normally the gallbladder is not palpable. If markedly distended it is palpable at the tip of the ninth costal cartilage on the right side.

49. a) **TRUE**   This enables the gallbladder to contract.
    b) **FALSE**   The main stimulus is hormonal.
    c) **FALSE**   The gallbladder is also supplied by arteries entering it directly from the liver.
    d) **FALSE**   The sphincter of Oddi in the duodenum regulates the flow of bile.
    e) **TRUE**   Cholecystokinin also stimulates the pancreas and relaxes the sphincter of Oddi.

The Digestive System

DEVELOPMENT OF THE GUT AND PERITONEAL CAVITY

True/False

50. Concerning the foregut:
    a) the stomach is a derivative
    b) it is supplied by the coeliac trunk
    c) it rotates 90° during development
    d) it communicates with the yolk sac
    e) it is attached to the ventral mesentery

51. The ventral mesentery contributes to
    a) the gastrosplenic ligament
    b) the lesser omentum
    c) the coronary ligament
    d) the falciform ligament
    e) the left triangular ligament

52. Concerning the midgut:
    a) the left colic flexure is a derivative
    b) it is supplied by the superior mesenteric artery
    c) it is connected to the yolk sac by the vitello-intestinal duct
    d) the caecum is derived from the distal limb of the loop
    e) the distal limb lies dorsal to the proximal limb after returning to the abdominal cavity from the umbilical cord

53. Concerning the hindgut:
    a) the part of the gut from the left colic flexure to the anal orifice is derived from it
    b) it contributes to the urinary bladder, urethra and vagina
    c) it is supplied by the inferior mesenteric artery
    d) it is connected to the umbilicus through the urachus
    e) the prostate gland is a derivative

The Digestive System

DEVELOPMENT OF THE GUT AND PERITONEAL CAVITY

50. a) **TRUE** The stomach appears in the fourth week of development.
    b) **TRUE**
    c) **TRUE** Rotation through 90° clockwise forms the lesser sac (omental bursa).
    d) **FALSE** It is the midgut that communicates with the yolk sac.
    e) **TRUE**

51. a) **FALSE** The gastrosplenic ligament derives from the dorsal mesentery.
    b) **TRUE**
    c) **TRUE**
    d) **TRUE**
    e) **TRUE**

52. a) **FALSE** The left colic flexure (splenic flexure) is derived from the hindgut.
    b) **TRUE**
    c) **TRUE** In the adult, the Meckel's diverticulum is a remnant of the vitello-intestinal duct.
    d) **TRUE** The caecal swelling is the last part of the midgut to re-enter the abdomen.
    e) **FALSE** The distal limb lies ventrally as it forms the large intestine.

53. a) **FALSE** The distal third of the transverse colon to the upper part of the anal canal is derived from the hindgut.
    b) **TRUE** The urorectal septum grows into the cloaca to separate the primitive urogenital sinus from the anorectal canal.
    c) **TRUE**
    d) **TRUE** The median umbilical ligament is a fibrous cord which is a remnant of the urachus (allantois).
    e) **TRUE** The glandular elements of the prostate develop from the epithelium of the prostatic urethra.

The Digestive System

54. **Regarding the ligaments of the liver:**
    a) the falciform ligament contains the ligamentum teres
    b) the ligamentum teres is the obliterated umbilical artery
    c) between the two layers of the coronary ligament is the bare area of the liver
    d) the left triangular ligament continues as the lesser omentum
    e) the coronary ligament ends as the right triangular ligament

55. **The lesser omentum**
    a) is attached to the porta hepatis
    b) contains the common bile duct, common hepatic artery and inferior vena cava
    c) has the common bile duct lying to the left of the common hepatic artery in the free border
    d) is attached to the gastroduodenal junction
    e) contains the left and right gastric arteries

56. **The following structures lie in the gastrosplenic ligament:**
    a) the short gastric arteries
    b) the splenic vein
    c) the common hepatic artery
    d) the tail of the pancreas
    e) the coeliac plexus

57. **The greater omentum**
    a) contains fat only in an obese person
    b) contains the left and right gastroepiploic arteries
    c) continues as the lesser omentum
    d) is continuous with the transverse mesocolon
    e) contains an extension of the lesser sac

198

The Digestive System

54. a) **TRUE** The ligamentum teres runs in the falciform ligament before reaching the liver.
    b) **FALSE** It is the remnant of the left umbilical vein.
    c) **TRUE** The bare area is bounded by the layers of the coronary ligament and the inferior vena cava.
    d) **TRUE** The left triangular ligament continues as the anterior layer of the lesser omentum.
    e) **TRUE**

55. a) **TRUE** It is also attached to the groove for the ligamentum venosum.
    b) **FALSE** It contains the common bile duct, common hepatic artery and portal vein.
    c) **FALSE** The common bile duct lies on the right; the portal vein lies posteriorly.
    d) **FALSE** The attachment extends from the abdominal oesophagus to the first inch of the duodenum.
    e) **TRUE** The two arteries run between the layers of the lesser omentum along the lesser curvature of the stomach.

56. a) **TRUE** Along with the left gastroepiploic artery. Both are branches of the splenic artery.
    b) **FALSE** The splenic vein is retroperitoneal except near the spleen where it lies in the lienorenal ligament.
    c) **FALSE** The common hepatic artery lies in the lesser omentum.
    d) **FALSE** The tail of the pancreas lies in the lienorenal ligament.
    e) **FALSE** The plexus surrounds the coeliac trunk and is retroperitoneal.

57. a) **FALSE** It is a fat store in all people.
    b) **TRUE** The arteries anastomose along the greater curvature of the stomach.
    c) **TRUE** The greater omentum splits to enclose the stomach and continues upward as the lesser omentum.
    d) **TRUE**
    e) **TRUE** As it folds back on itself, it encloses an extension of the lesser sac.

The Digestive System

58. **Regarding the parietal peritoneum of the anterior abdominal wall:**
    a) it is reflected onto the anterior surface of the urinary bladder
    b) the median umbilical fold is contributed to by the remnant of the urachus
    c) the medial umbilical fold is contributed to by the obliterated umbilical artery
    d) the lateral umbilical fold is contributed to by the inferior epigastric artery
    e) it is supplied by the intercostal nerves

59. **Regarding the pelvic peritoneum:**
    a) it is reflected from the upper third of the rectum to the posterior surface of the uterus
    b) the uterovesical pouch is at a higher level than the rectouterine pouch
    c) the rectouterine pouch is the most dependent part of the peritoneal cavity
    d) the posterior surface of the bladder is not covered by peritoneum
    e) the broad ligament contains the uterine tubes

The Digestive System

58. a) **FALSE** Only the superior surface of the bladder is covered by peritoneum.
    b) **TRUE** The median umbilical ligament, which produces the fold, is a remnant of the urachus.
    c) **TRUE**
    d) **TRUE** The artery arises from the external iliac artery and lies medial to the deep inguinal ring.
    e) **TRUE** The nerves supplying the abdominal wall also supply the parietal peritoneum.

59. a) **FALSE** It is reflected onto the posterior surface of the upper part of the vagina.
    b) **TRUE**
    c) **TRUE** The rectouterine pouch is also known as the pouch of Douglas and is about 5.5 cm above the anal margin.
    d) **TRUE** The posterior surface of the bladder is related either to the seminal vesicles and ductus deferens or to the vagina.
    e) **TRUE** However, the ovaries project posteriorly from the broad ligament.

The Digestive System

Picture questions

Identify the numbered structures in the following illustrations from the choices given

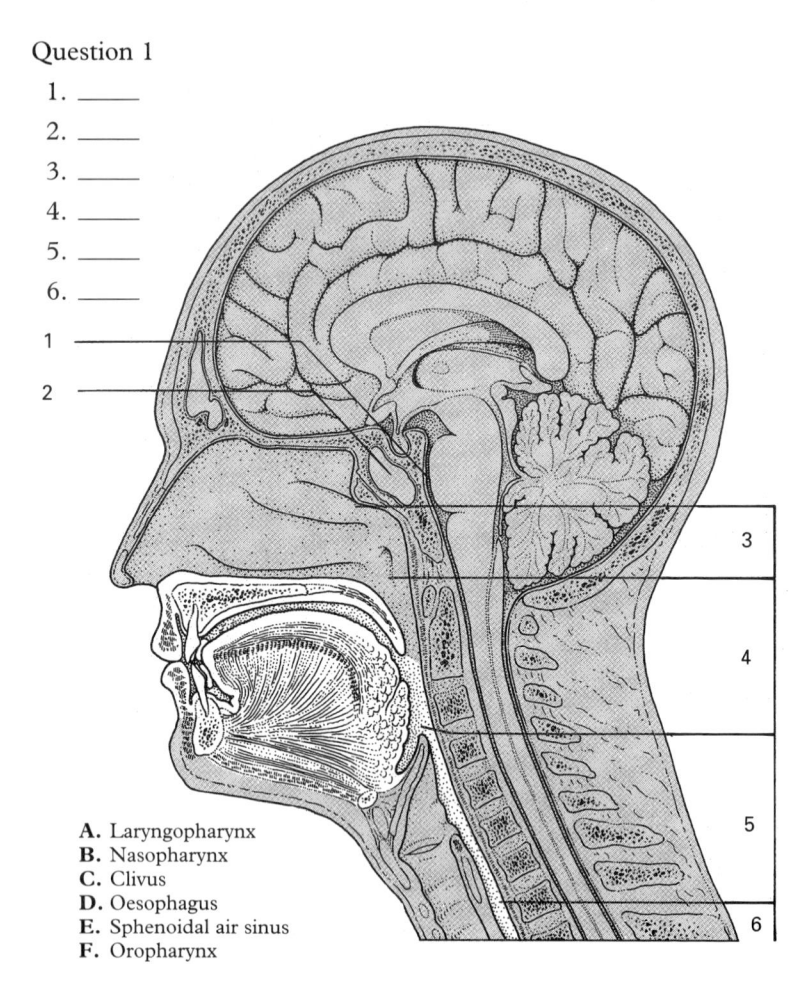

Question 1
1. ____
2. ____
3. ____
4. ____
5. ____
6. ____

A. Laryngopharynx
B. Nasopharynx
C. Clivus
D. Oesophagus
E. Sphenoidal air sinus
F. Oropharynx

The Digestive System

Question 2
1. ___
2. ___
3. ___
4. ___
5. ___
6. ___
7. ___

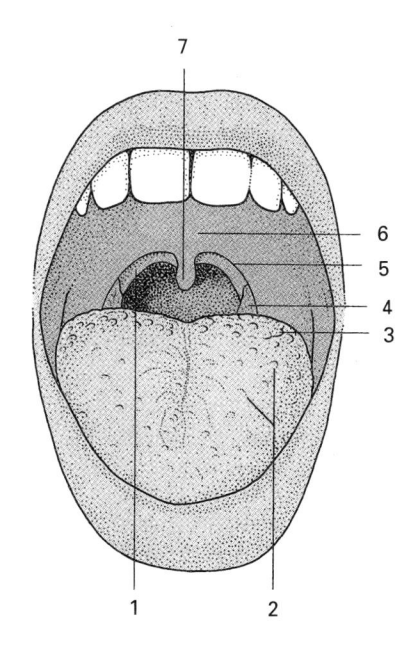

A. Uvula
B. Palatopharyngeal fold
C. Valate papilla
D. Palatine tonsil
E. Palatoglossal fold
F. Fungiform papillae
G. Soft palate

Question 3
1. ___
2. ___
3. ___
4. ___
5. ___
6. ___

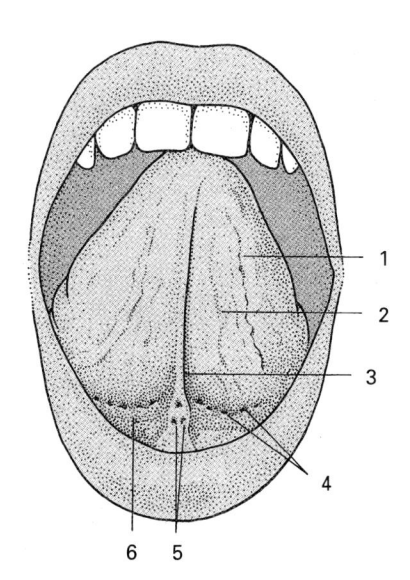

A. Fimbriated fold
B. Submandibular ducts
C. Frenulum
D. Deep lingual vein
E. Sublingual fold
F. Sublingual ducts

Answers on page 218   203

The Digestive System

Question 4

1. ____
2. ____
3. ____
4. ____
5. ____
6. ____
7. ____
8. ____
9. ____
10. ____
11. ____
12. ____
13. ____
14. ____

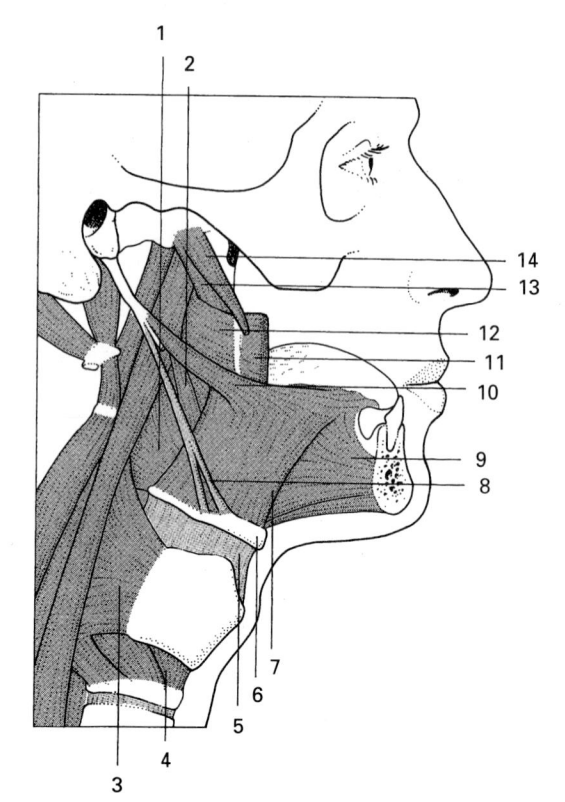

A. Inferior constrictor
B. Middle constrictor
C. Thyrohyoid membrane
D. Superior constrictor
E. Tensor palatini
F. Levator palatini
G. Cricothyroid
H. Stylohyoid ligament
I. Styloglossus
J. Hyoid
K. Buccinator
L. Hyoglossus
M. Genioglossus
N. Styloglossus

The Digestive System

Question 5
1. ____
2. ____
3. ____
4. ____
5. ____
6. ____
7. ____
8. ____
9. ____

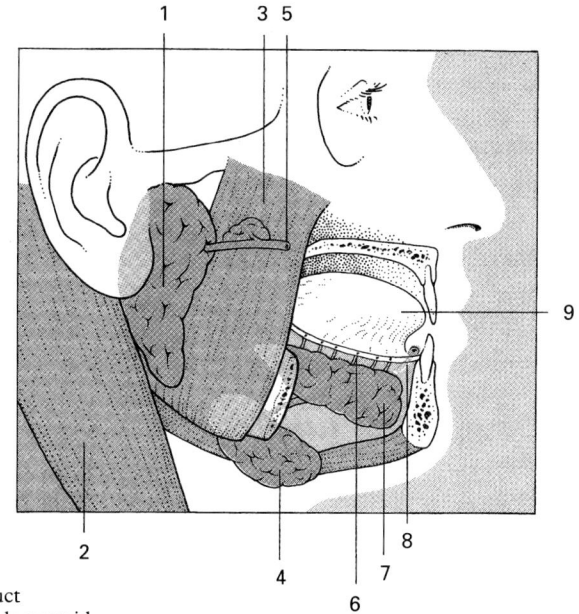

A. Parotid duct
B. Sternocleidomastoid
C. Tongue
D. Sublingual ducts
E. Submandibular gland
F. Sublingual gland
G. Masseter
H. Parotid gland
I. Submandibular duct

The Digestive System

Question 6
1. ___
2. ___
3. ___
4. ___
5. ___
6. ___
7. ___
8. ___
9. ___
10. ___
11. ___

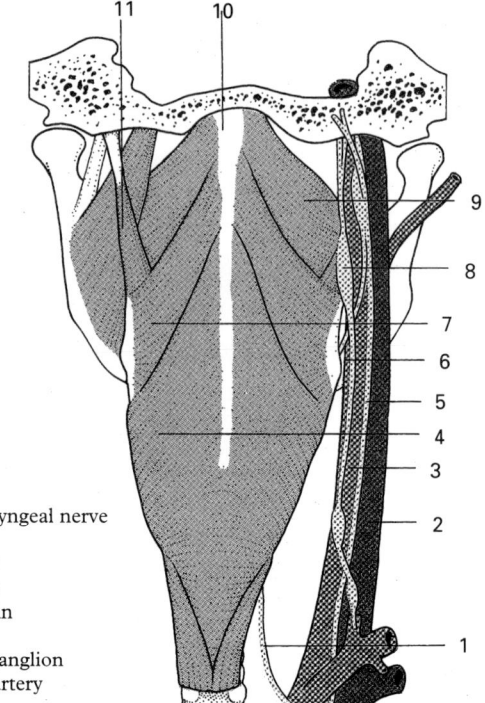

A. Right recurrent laryngeal nerve
B. Stylopharyngeus
C. Sympathetic trunk
D. Middle constrictor
E. Internal jugular vein
F. Pharyngeal raphe
G. Superior cervical ganglion
H. Common carotid artery
I. Vagus nerve
J. Inferior constrictor
K. Superior constrictor

The Digestive System

Question 7
1. ____
2. ____
3. ____
4. ____
5. ____
6. ____
7. ____
8. ____
9. ____
10. ____
11. ____

A. Epiglottis
B. Laryngeal inlet
C. Piriform fossa
D. Superior constrictor
E. Tongue showing lingual tonsil
F. Eustachian tube
G. Palatine tonsil
H. Uvula
I. Soft palate
J. Nasal cavity
K. Nasopharynx

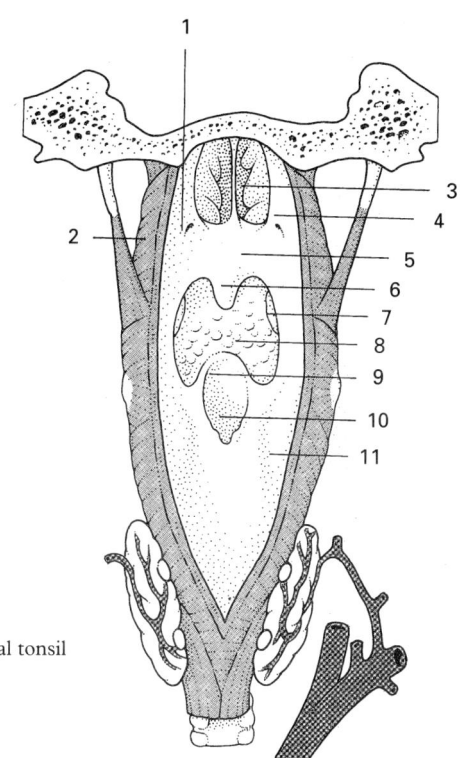

The Digestive System

Question 8

1. ___
2. ___
3. ___
4. ___
5. ___
6. ___
7. ___
8. ___
9. ___
10. ___
11. ___
12. ___
13. ___
14. ___
15. ___

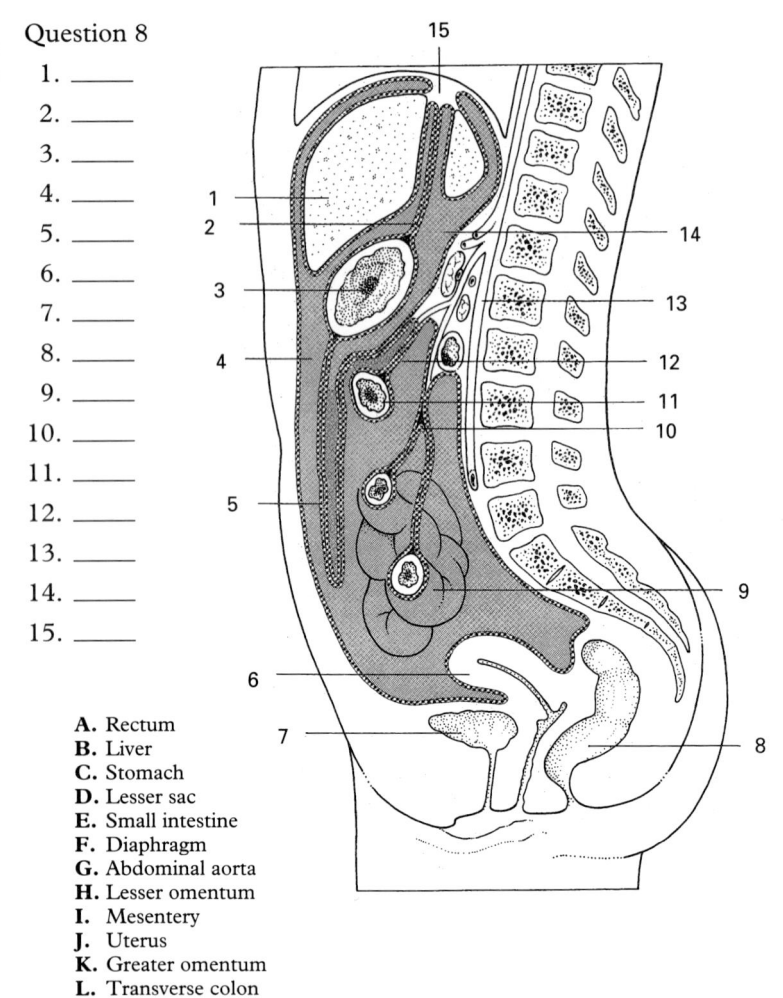

A. Rectum
B. Liver
C. Stomach
D. Lesser sac
E. Small intestine
F. Diaphragm
G. Abdominal aorta
H. Lesser omentum
I. Mesentery
J. Uterus
K. Greater omentum
L. Transverse colon
M. Transverse mesocolon
N. Greater sac
O. Urinary bladder

The Digestive System

Question 9
1. ____
2. ____
3. ____
4. ____
5. ____
6. ____
7. ____
8. ____
9. ____
10. ____

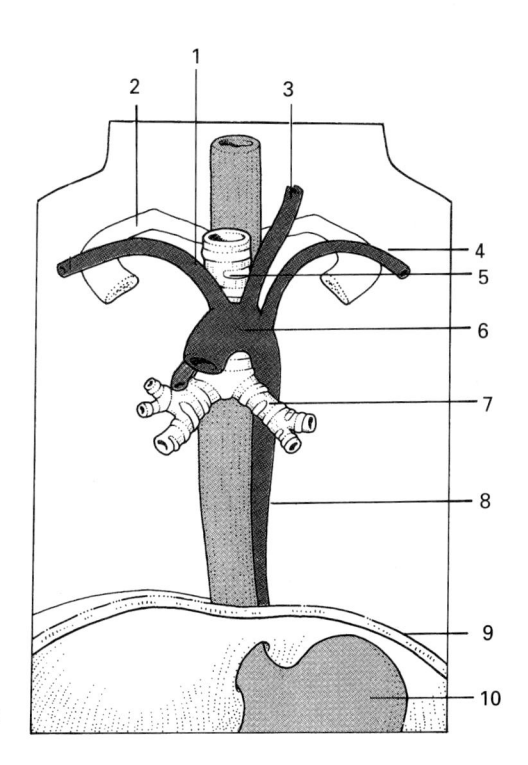

A. First rib
B. Left common carotid artery
C. Diaphragm
D. Trachea
E. Arch of aorta
F. Left bronchus
G. Left subclavian artery
H. Descending aorta
I. Brachiocephalic artery
J. Stomach

The Digestive System

Question 10
1. ____
2. ____
3. ____
4. ____
5. ____
6. ____
7. ____
8. ____
9. ____
10. ____
11. ____
12. ____

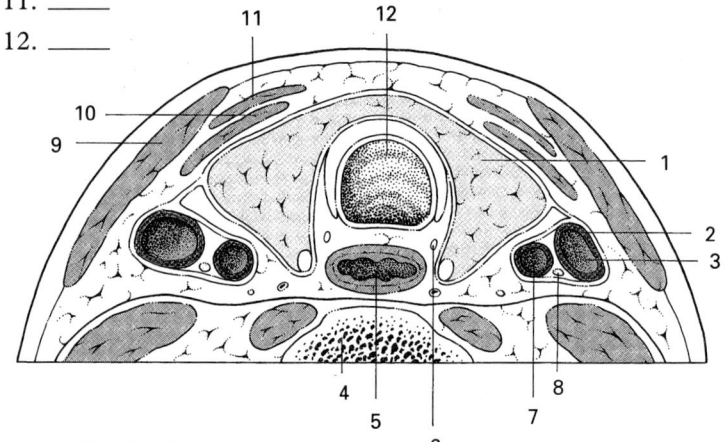

A. Vertebra C7
B. Common carotid artery
C. Oesophagus
D. Vagus nerve
E. Sternothyroid
F. Thyroid gland
G. Trachea
H. Internal jugular vein
I. Sternohyoid
J. Carotid sheath
K. Recurrent laryngeal nerve
L. Sternomastoid

210

The Digestive System

Question 11

1. ___
2. ___
3. ___
4. ___
5. ___
6. ___
7. ___
8. ___
9. ___
10. ___
11. ___
12. ___
13. ___
14. ___

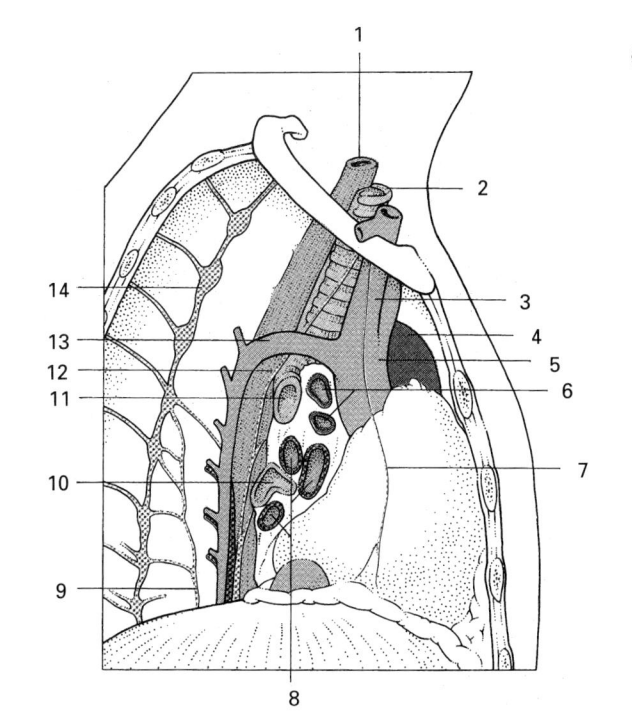

A. Sympathetic trunk
B. Azygos vein
C. Superior lobe bronchus
D. Greater splanchnic nerve
E. Pulmonary artery
F. Right phrenic nerve
G. Right brachiocephalic vein
H. Oesophagus
I. Arch of aorta
J. Pulmonary veins
K. Right vagus
L. Right bronchus
M. Trachea
N. Superior vena cava

Answers on pages 220 and 221 211

The Digestive System

Question 12
1. ____
2. ____
3. ____
4. ____

   A. Lesser curvature
   B. Duodenal cap
   C. Jejunum
   D. Greater curvature

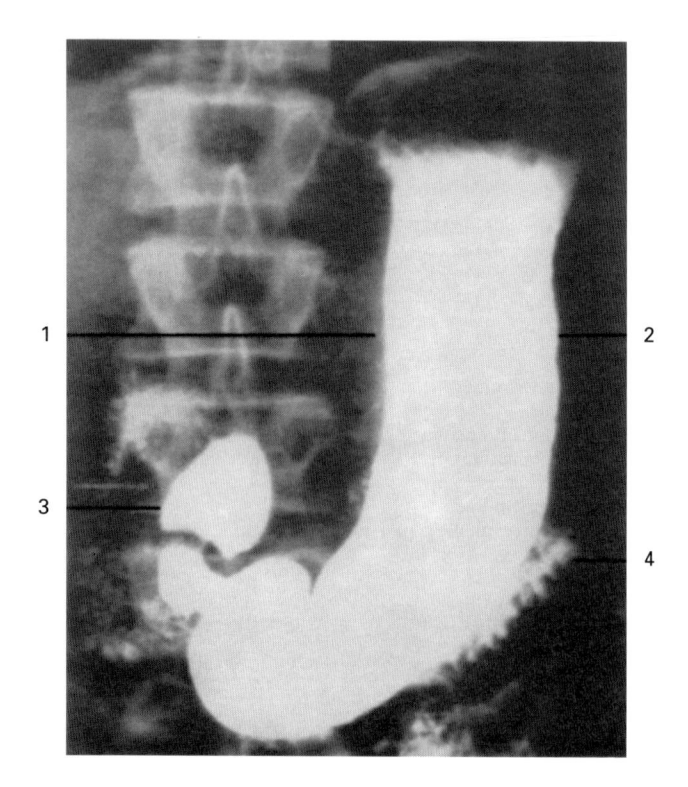

The Digestive System

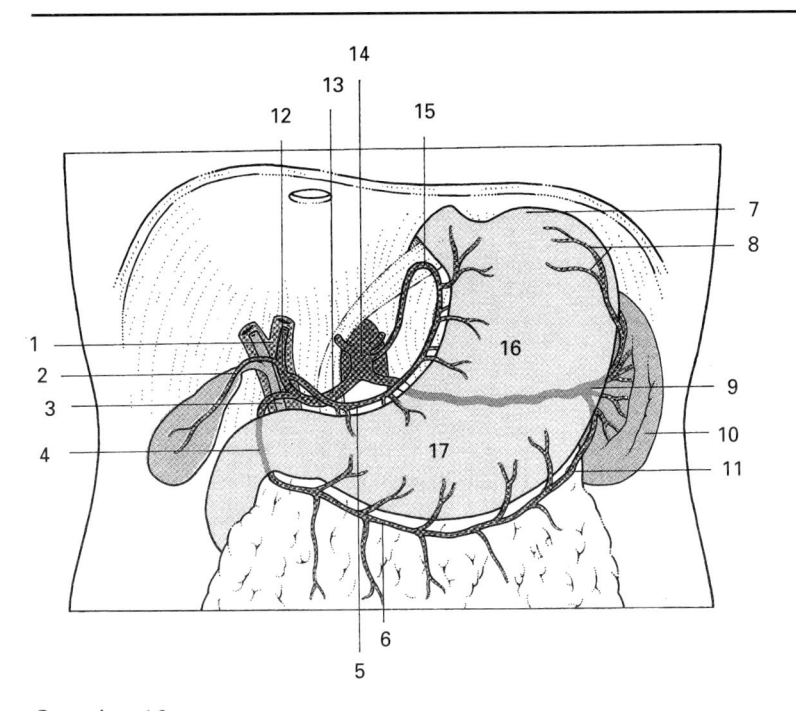

Question 13

1. ____
2. ____
3. ____
4. ____
5. ____
6. ____
7. ____
8. ____
9. ____
10. ____
11. ____
12. ____
13. ____
14. ____
15. ____
16. ____
17. ____

A. Hepatic portal vein
B. Common bile duct
C. Right gastric artery
D. Splenic artery
E. Left gastroepiploic artery
F. Hepatic artery
G. Coeliac trunk
H. Body of stomach
I. Cystic artery
J. Pyloric part of stomach
K. Right gastroepiploic artery
L. Gastroduodenal artery
M. Fundus of stomach
N. Spleen
O. Short gastric arteries
P. Common hepatic artery
Q. Left gastric artery

Answers on page 221   213

The Digestive System

Question 14
1. ___
2. ___
3. ___
4. ___
5. ___
6. ___
7. ___
8. ___
9. ___
10. ___
11. ___
12. ___
13. ___

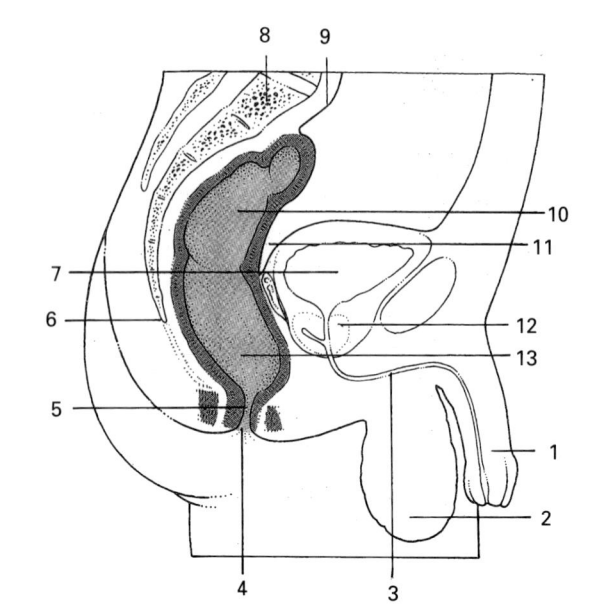

A. Coccyx
B. Penis
C. Peritoneum
D. Bladder
E. Urethra
F. Rectal ampulla
G. Prostate
H. Rectovesical pouch
I. Anal canal
J. Sacrum
K. Rectum
L. Anus
M. Scrotum

The Digestive System

Question 15
1. ___
2. ___
3. ___
4. ___
5. ___
6. ___
7. ___
8. ___
9. ___
10. ___
11. ___
12. ___

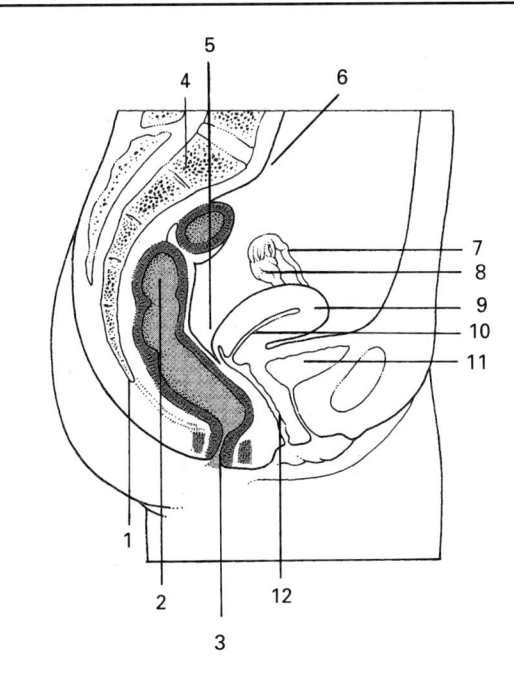

A. Ovary
B. Bladder
C. Peritoneum
D. Uterine tube
E. Sacrum
F. Rectouterine pouch
G. Vagina
H. Anal canal
I. Uterus
J. Coccyx
K. Rectum
L. Broad ligament (cut)

Answers on page 222   215

The Digestive System

Question 16
1. ____
2. ____
3. ____
4. ____
5. ____
6. ____
7. ____
8. ____
9. ____
10. ____
11. ____
12. ____
13. ____
14. ____
15. ____
16. ____
17. ____
18. ____

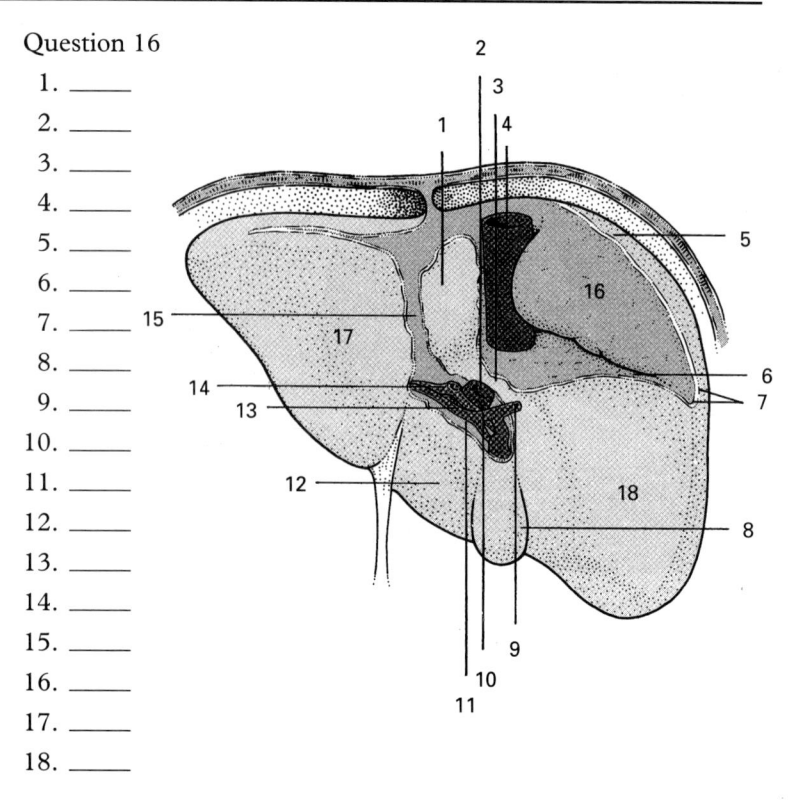

A. Lesser omentum (cut) in the fissure for ligamentum venosum
B. Right lobe
C. Portal vein
D. Gallbladder
E. Common hepatic duct
F. Porta hepatis
G. Hepatic artery
H. Caudate lobe
I. Left hepatic duct
J. Inferior vena cava
K. Quadrate lobe
L. Caudate process
M. Bare area
N. Right triangular ligament
O. Left lobe
P. Superior layer of coronary ligament (cut)
Q. Common bile duct
R. Inferior layer of coronary ligament (cut)

The Digestive System

Question 17
1. ____
2. ____
3. ____
4. ____
5. ____
6. ____
7. ____
8. ____
9. ____
10. ____
11. ____
12. ____
13. ____
14. ____
15. ____
16. ____
17. ____

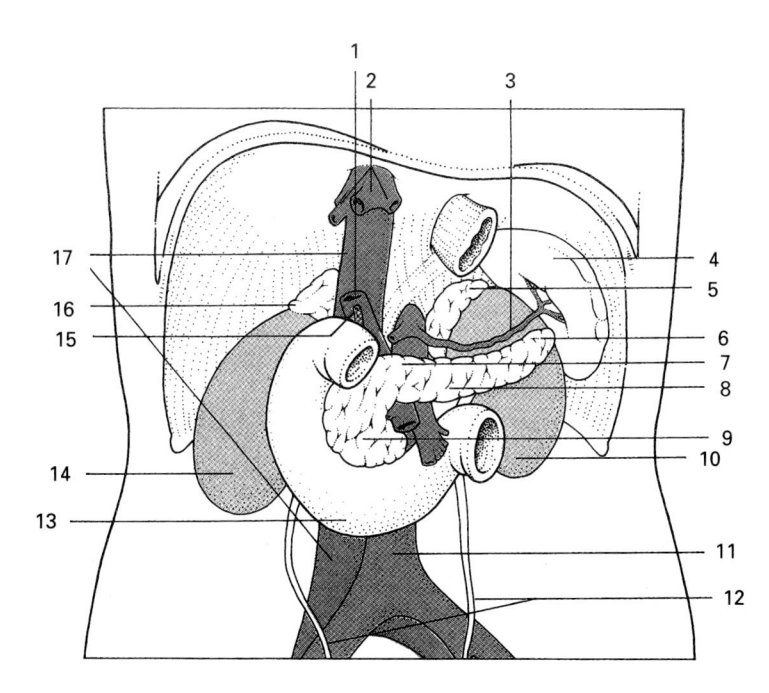

A. Neck of pancreas
B. Aorta
C. Head of pancreas
D. Inferior vena cava
E. Ureters
F. Hepatic veins
G. Body of pancreas
H. Tail of pancreas
I. Splenic artery
J. Right suprarenal gland
K. Common bile duct
L. Duodenum
M. Portal vein
N. Right kidney
O. Left kidney
P. Spleen
Q. Left suprarenal gland

Answers on page 223

The Digestive System

A Picture questions

Question 1
1. **C** Clivus
2. **E** Sphenoidal air sinus
3. **B** Nasopharynx
4. **F** Oropharynx
5. **A** Laryngopharynx
6. **D** Oesophagus

Question 2
1. **B** Palatopharyngeal fold
2. **F** Fungiform papillae
3. **C** Valate papilla
4. **D** Palatine tonsil
5. **E** Palatoglossal fold
6. **G** Soft palate
7. **A** Uvula

Question 3
1. **A** Fimbriated fold
2. **D** Deep lingual vein
3. **C** Frenulum
4. **F** Sublingual ducts
5. **B** Submandibular ducts
6. **E** Sublingual fold

Question 4
1. **B** Middle constrictor
2. **I** Styloglossus
3. **A** Inferior constrictor
4. **G** Cricothyroid
5. **C** Thyrohyoid membrane
6. **J** Hyoid
7. **L** Hyoglossus
8. **H** Stylohyoid ligament
9. **M** Genioglossus
10. **N** Styloglossus
11. **K** Buccinator
12. **D** Superior constrictor
13. **F** Levator palatini
14. **E** Tensor palatini

The Digestive System

Question 5
1. **H** Parotid gland
2. **B** Sternocleidomastoid
3. **G** Masseter
4. **E** Submandibular gland
5. **A** Parotid duct
6. **D** Sublingual ducts
7. **F** Sublingual gland
8. **I** Submandibular duct
9. **C** Tongue

Question 6
1. **A** Right recurrent laryngeal nerve
2. **E** Internal jugular vein
3. **H** Common carotid artery
4. **J** Inferior constrictor
5. **I** Vagus nerve
6. **C** Sympathetic trunk
7. **D** Middle constrictor
8. **G** Superior cervical ganglion
9. **K** Superior constrictor
10. **F** Pharyngeal raphe
11. **B** Stylopharyngeus

Question 7
1. **F** Eustachian tube
2. **D** Superior constrictor
3. **J** Nasal cavity
4. **K** Nasopharynx
5. **I** Soft palate
6. **H** Uvula
7. **G** Palatine tonsil
8. **E** Tongue showing lingual tonsil
9. **A** Epiglottis
10. **B** Laryngeal inlet
11. **C** Piriform fossa

The Digestive System

Question 8
1. **B** Liver
2. **H** Lesser omentum
3. **C** Stomach
4. **N** Greater sac
5. **K** Greater omentum
6. **J** Uterus
7. **O** Urinary bladder
8. **A** Rectum
9. **E** Small intestine
10. **I** Mesentery
11. **L** Transverse colon
12. **M** Transverse mesocolon
13. **G** Abdominal aorta
14. **D** Lesser sac
15. **F** Diaphragm

Question 9
1. **I** Brachiocephalic artery
2. **A** First rib
3. **B** Left common carotid artery
4. **G** Left subclavian artery
5. **D** Trachea
6. **E** Arch of aorta
7. **F** Left bronchus
8. **H** Descending aorta
9. **C** Diaphragm
10. **J** Stomach

Question 10
1. **F** Thyroid gland
2. **J** Carotid sheath
3. **H** Internal jugular vein
4. **A** Vertebra C7
5. **C** Oesophagus
6. **K** Recurrent laryngeal nerve
7. **B** Common carotid artery
8. **D** Vagus nerve
9. **L** Sternomastoid
10. **E** Sternothyroid
11. **I** Sternohyoid
12. **G** Trachea

The Digestive System

Question 11
1. **H** Oesophagus
2. **M** Trachea
3. **G** Right brachiocephalic vein
4. **I** Arch of aorta
5. **N** Superior vena cava
6. **E** Pulmonary artery
7. **F** Right phrenic nerve
8. **J** Pulmonary veins
9. **D** Greater splanchnic nerve
10. **L** Right bronchus
11. **C** Superior lobe bronchus
12. **K** Right vagus
13. **B** Azygos vein
14. **A** Sympathetic trunk

Question 12
1. **A** Lesser curvature
2. **D** Greater curvature
3. **B** Duodenal cap
4. **C** Jejunum

Question 13
1. **A** Hepatic portal vein
2. **I** Cystic artery
3. **B** Common bile duct
4. **L** Gastroduodenal artery
5. **C** Right gastric artery
6. **K** Right gastroepiploic artery
7. **M** Fundus of stomach
8. **O** Short gastric arteries
9. **D** Splenic artery
10. **N** Spleen
11. **E** Left gastroepiploic artery
12. **F** Hepatic artery
13. **P** Common hepatic artery
14. **G** Coeliac trunk
15. **Q** Left gastric artery
16. **H** Body of stomach
17. **J** Pyloric part of stomach

The Digestive System

Question 14
1. **B** Penis
2. **M** Scrotum
3. **E** Urethra
4. **L** Anus
5. **I** Anal canal
6. **A** Coccyx
7. **D** Bladder
8. **J** Sacrum
9. **C** Peritoneum
10. **K** Rectum
11. **H** Rectovesical pouch
12. **G** Prostate
13. **F** Rectal ampulla

Question 15
1. **J** Coccyx
2. **K** Rectum
3. **H** Anal canal
4. **E** Sacrum
5. **F** Rectouterine pouch
6. **C** Peritoneum
7. **D** Uterine tube
8. **A** Ovary
9. **I** Uterus
10. **L** Broad ligament (cut)
11. **B** Bladder
12. **G** Vagina

The Digestive System

Question 16
1. **H** Caudate lobe
2. **C** Portal vein
3. **L** Caudate process
4. **J** Inferior vena cava
5. **P** Superior layer of coronary ligament (cut)
6. **R** Inferior layer of coronary ligament (cut)
7. **N** Right triangular ligament
8. **D** Gallbladder
9. **Q** Common bile duct
10. **E** Common hepatic duct
11. **F** Porta hepatis
12. **K** Quadrate lobe
13. **I** Left hepatic duct
14. **G** Hepatic artery
15. **A** Lesser omentum (cut) in fissure for ligamentum venosum
16. **M** Bare area
17. **O** Left lobe
18. **B** Right lobe

Question 17
1. **M** Portal vein
2. **F** Hepatic veins
3. **I** Splenic artery
4. **P** Spleen
5. **Q** Left suprarenal gland
6. **H** Tail of pancreas
7. **A** Neck of pancreas
8. **G** Body of pancreas
9. **C** Head of pancreas
10. **O** Left kidney
11. **B** Aorta
12. **E** Ureters
13. **L** Duodenum
14. **N** Right kidney
15. **K** Common bile duct
16. **J** Right suprarenal gland
17. **D** Inferior vena cava

The Digestive System

Clinical problems

1. A middle-aged man with a long history of alcoholism and liver disease is brought to hospital after vomiting a large amount of blood. What might have caused the bleeding?

2. A carcinoma of the rectum if left undiagnosed can penetrate into adjoining structures. What are the structures it can spread locally into?

3. A 57-year-old female, a heavy smoker, attended her doctor's surgery complaining of difficulty in swallowing and a change in her voice. Clinical examination revealed that she had an ulcer in the posterior third of her tongue. A biopsy was taken later which showed that the ulcer was malignant. To which lymph node groups will it spread? To what structures may it spread locally? Which nerve will transmit pain from this part of the tongue?

4. Acute appendicitis is one of the commonest acute abdominal emergencies. What is the surface marking of the appendix? What are the commonest positions of the appendix? How do you identify the root of the appendix at operation?

5. How can a large gallstone obstruct the ileum?

The Digestive System

A Clinical problems

1. Intake of a large amount of alcohol for a long period can produce cirrhosis of the liver. This involves scarring and fibrosis of the liver obstructing the branches of the portal vein. Portal hypertension will result. Enlargement of portosystemic anastomoses at the lower end of the oesophagus gives rise to oesophageal varices which burst, resulting in haematemesis (vomiting of blood).

2. A carcinoma of the rectum in the male can spread anteriorly into the prostate, seminal vesicles and urinary bladder. In the female, the vagina and uterus may be invaded. The carcinoma can spread laterally into the ureter, and posteriorly into the sacrum and the sacral plexus of nerves.

3. From the posterior third of the tongue, a malignant tumour may spread bilaterally into the upper deep cervical lymph nodes. It can spread locally into a number of adjoining structures, viz. the tonsil, side of the pharynx, cervical spine, soft palate, epiglottis and downwards into the larynx. Pain from the posterior third of the tongue is transmitted by the glossopharyngeal nerve.

4. Surface marking of the appendix is the McBurney's point which lies at the junction between the lower and middle third of a line joining the umbilicus to the right anterior superior iliac spine. The appendix is commonly retrocaecal (behind the caecum). It can be pelvic, crossing the brim of the pelvis, paracaecal, pre-ileal or post-ileal. The root of the appendix is at the point where the three taeniae coli meet and it can thus be found by tracing the taeniae coli inferiorly.

5. A large gallstone cannot pass through the bile duct and enter the duodenum. The gallbladder lies in the front of the first and second parts of the duodenum and the stone can ulcerate into it through its wall. If it is large enough, it can cause duodenal obstruction. If not, the stone may pass to the ileum and may block the narrowest part of the small intestine which is about 60 cm from the ileocaecal junction, giving rise to a condition known as 'gallstone ileus'.

The Respiratory System

The Respiratory System

THE RESPIRATORY SYSTEM

True/False

1. **Concerning the nasal cavity:**
   a) the inferior meatus lies below the inferior concha
   b) the most expanded part is the superior meatus
   c) the nasolacrimal duct opens into the middle meatus
   d) it is supplied entirely by branches of the external carotid artery
   e) the anterior ethmoidal nerve supplies the septum

2. **With regard to the paranasal sinuses:**
   a) the frontal and ethmoidal sinuses are closely related to the frontal lobe of the brain
   b) the maxillary sinus has an opening in its most dependent part
   c) the maxillary sinus is closely related to the upper molar teeth
   d) carcinoma of the maxillary sinus may spread into the orbit
   e) the sphenoidal sinus is closely related to the pituitary gland

3. **Concerning the nasopharynx:**
   a) the auditory (eustachian) tube opens on the lateral wall
   b) the opening of the auditory tube is bounded behind by the tubal elevation
   c) adenoids can cause deafness and middle ear infection
   d) the pharyngeal recess lies in front of the eustachian tube
   e) it is innervated by the glossopharyngeal nerve

The Respiratory System

1. a) **TRUE** Each meatus lies below the respective concha.
   b) **FALSE** The inferior meatus is the largest. Hence nasal endotracheal tubes are passed through the inferior meatus.
   c) **FALSE** It opens into the inferior meatus.
   d) **FALSE** The anterior ethmoidal artery is a branch of the ophthalmic artery given off from the internal carotid.
   e) **TRUE** It also supplies the lateral wall and becomes the external nasal nerve. It is a branch of the nasociliary branch of the ophthalmic division of the trigeminal nerve.

2. a) **TRUE** These sinuses lie in the frontal bone and ethmoidal bone respectively. Infection or tumour from the sinuses can spread into the brain.
   b) **FALSE** The opening of the maxillary sinus is towards the upper part of its medial wall and is inefficiently placed for drainage.
   c) **TRUE** A bad extraction of the tooth may cause an antro-oral fistula.
   d) **TRUE** The orbit lies above the sinus.
   e) **TRUE** The pituitary gland lies above the sinus. The pituitary can be surgically approached through the trans-sphenoidal route.

3. a) **TRUE** The auditory tube connects the nasopharynx and the middle ear.
   b) **TRUE** This prominence is used as a landmark in identifying the opening during catheterisation of the eustachian tube.
   c) **TRUE** Enlargement of the nasopharyngeal tonsil (adenoids) will block the eustachian tube, causing deafness. It blocks the nasopharynx causing mouth-breathing. Infection usually spreads to the middle ear through the eustachian tube.
   d) **FALSE** The recess is the area behind the tubal elevation and hence behind the tube.
   e) **FALSE** The sensory innervation is through branches of the maxillary nerve.

The Respiratory System

4. **The following statements about the laryngopharynx are true:**
   a) the larynx bulges into it
   b) the piriform fossa is the space behind the larynx
   c) the mucosa is innervated by the recurrent laryngeal nerve
   d) sharp foreign bodies, such as fish bones, may get lodged in the piriform fossa
   e) the internal laryngeal nerve is embedded in the muscle wall

5. **Concerning the larynx:**
   a) the vocal cords are tensed by the cricothyroid muscles
   b) the cricothyroid muscle is supplied by the recurrent laryngeal nerve
   c) the rima glottidis is opened by the lateral cricoarytenoid muscles
   d) the posterior cricoarytenoid muscles are attached to the muscular process of the arytenoid cartilage
   e) the whole laryngeal mucosa is covered by respiratory epithelium

6. **The recurrent laryngeal nerve is intimately related to the following structures:**
   a) the ligamentum arteriosum
   b) the oesophagus
   c) the inferior thyroid artery
   d) the internal carotid artery
   e) the subclavian artery

7. **The superior laryngeal nerve**
   a) passes between the internal carotid artery and the external carotid artery
   b) has cells of origin in the medulla oblongata
   c) supplies the middle constrictor
   d) gives a branch to and lies in the submucosa of the piriform fossa
   e) is purely motor

The Respiratory System

4. a) **TRUE**
   b) **FALSE** It is the space on either side of the larynx.
   c) **FALSE** Sensory innervation is by the internal laryngeal nerve.
   d) **TRUE** And their removal may damage the internal laryngeal nerve.
   e) **FALSE** The nerve lies just under the mucosa and can be blocked by topical application of anaesthetic agents.

5. a) **FALSE** The cords are lengthened by the cricothyroids.
   b) **FALSE** It is supplied by the external laryngeal branch of the superior laryngeal nerve.
   c) **FALSE** The posterior cricoarytenoids abduct the cords.
   d) **TRUE** And also to the lamina of the cricoid.
   e) **FALSE** The vocal cords are covered by stratified squamous epithelium.

6. a) **TRUE** The left nerve is given off from the vagus at this level and it winds round the ligament.
   b) **TRUE** It lies in the groove between the trachea and the oesophagus.
   c) **TRUE** The nerve crosses the artery near the lower pole of the thyroid gland.
   d) **FALSE**
   e) **TRUE** The right nerve winds round this artery.

7. a) **FALSE** It passes deep to both the carotids.
   b) **TRUE** The cells of origin of the fibres of the external laryngeal nerve are in the nucleus ambiguus.
   c) **FALSE** All the constrictors are supplied by the pharyngeal branch of the vagus.
   d) **TRUE** This branch is the internal laryngeal nerve.
   e) **FALSE** The internal laryngeal branch is sensory.

The Respiratory System

8. **The recurrent laryngeal nerve**
   a) carries the sensory supply to the whole larynx
   b) supplies the mucosa below the vocal cords
   c) supplies all the intrinsic muscles of the larynx except thyroarytenoid
   d) supplies all the intrinsic muscles of the larynx except cricothyroid
   e) supplies the trachea

9. **The posterior cricoarytenoid muscle**
   a) is attached to the lamina of the thyroid cartilage
   b) is the only abductor of the vocal cords
   c) is attached to the muscular process of the arytenoid cartilage
   d) forms part of the anterior wall of the laryngopharynx
   e) is supplied by the superior laryngeal nerve

10. **In the living body, the trachea**
    a) lies in the midline in the thoracic inlet
    b) moves down with inspiration
    c) divides in the posterior mediastinum
    d) lies anterior to the oesophagus throughout its course
    e) is lined by stratified squamous epithelium

11. **The trachea**
    a) begins at the level of the sixth cervical vertebra
    b) contains incomplete rings of fibrocartilage
    c) obtains a blood supply from the inferior thyroid artery
    d) contains longitudinal muscle fibres in its posterior wall
    e) develops as an outgrowth from the primitive oesophagus

The Respiratory System

8. a) **FALSE** The part above the vocal cords receives its sensory supply from the internal laryngeal nerve.
   b) **TRUE**
   c) **FALSE** Thyroarytenoid is supplied by the recurrent laryngeal nerve.
   d) **TRUE** Cricothyroid is supplied by the external laryngeal nerve.
   e) **TRUE**

9. a) **FALSE** It is attached to the lamina of the cricoid cartilage.
   b) **TRUE**
   c) **TRUE**
   d) **TRUE**
   e) **FALSE** It is supplied by the recurrent laryngeal nerve.

10. a) **TRUE**
    b) **TRUE** It descends by about 5 cm.
    c) **TRUE** In the living, the division is below the level of the sternal angle.
    d) **TRUE**
    e) **FALSE** It is lined by pseudostratified ciliated columnar epithelium (respiratory epithelium).

11. a) **TRUE** Both the trachea and the oesophagus begin at this level.
    b) **FALSE** It contains incomplete rings of hyaline cartilage.
    c) **TRUE** Bronchial arteries also supply the trachea.
    d) **TRUE** This is the trachealis muscle (nonstriated); it allows changes in diameter of the lumen, as in coughing.
    e) **TRUE** Developmental anomalies may result in a tracheo-oesophageal fistula.

The Respiratory System

12. **The left main bronchus**
    a) is about 5 cm in length
    b) is more in line with the trachea than is the right main bronchus
    c) is slightly narrower than the right main bronchus
    d) gives direct origin to the lingular bronchus
    e) lies in front of the oesophagus

13. **The right main bronchus**
    a) is shorter than the left main bronchus
    b) is narrower than the left main bronchus
    c) gives off all its branches inside the lung
    d) is enclosed by complete cartilaginous rings
    e) is closely related to the azygos vein

14. **In the root of the right lung**
    a) the upper lobe bronchus is superiorly placed
    b) the azygos vein is a close relation
    c) the pulmonary veins are anteriorly placed
    d) the main bronchus is the most anterior structure
    e) the phrenic nerve lies behind

15. **The root of the left lung**
    a) perforates the mediastinal pleura
    b) is closely related to the arch of the aorta
    c) contains lymph vessels but no nodes
    d) contains the main bronchus posteriorly
    e) contains bronchial arteries which are branches of the descending aorta

The Respiratory System

12. a) **TRUE**
    b) **FALSE** The right main bronchus is more vertical.
    c) **TRUE**
    d) **FALSE** The lingular bronchus is a branch of the superior lobar bronchus.
    e) **TRUE**

13. a) **TRUE** It gives off its upper lobe bronchus 2.5 cm below the bifurcation of the trachea.
    b) **FALSE**
    c) **FALSE** The upper lobe bronchus is given off outside the lung.
    d) **FALSE** The arrangement of cartilage is similar to that of the trachea (incomplete rings bridged by smooth muscle).
    e) **TRUE**

14. a) **TRUE**
    b) **TRUE** The vein hooks over the upper part of the right lung root.
    c) **TRUE**
    d) **FALSE** The bronchus is posterior.
    e) **FALSE** The nerve is in front of the root of the lung; the vagus lies behind.

15. a) **FALSE** The pleura forms a sleeve around the roots of the lungs and contributes to the pulmonary ligaments.
    b) **TRUE** The left lung root lies below the arch of the aorta.
    c) **FALSE** It contains the hilar lymph nodes which drain lymph from the lung into the tracheobronchial lymph nodes.
    d) **TRUE**
    e) **TRUE**

The Respiratory System

16. **Regarding the right lung:**
    a) the apex does not extend above the clavicle
    b) the azygos vein arches over its root
    c) the horizontal fissure lies along the sixth costal cartilage
    d) two bronchi enter its hilum
    e) it is related to the upper part of the right lobe of the liver

17. **Concerning the lungs:**
    a) each bronchopulmonary segment is ventilated by a tertiary bronchus
    b) the bronchus of the apical segment of the lower lobe passes anteriorly
    c) the epithelium is pseudostratified ciliated columnar throughout
    d) the terminal bronchioles are distal to the respiratory bronchioles
    e) mucous glands or cells are not seen in the alveolar sacs

18. **The pleura**
    a) has the same surface markings as the lungs
    b) is wholly innervated by both the intercostal and phrenic nerves
    c) does not extend into the fissures of the lung
    d) extends upwards into the neck above the medial third of the clavicle
    e) is grooved in its uppermost part by the subclavian artery

19. **In laboured breathing during the inspiratory phase, the following muscles may be noticeably active:**
    a) pectoralis major
    b) serratus anterior
    c) sternocleidomastoid
    d) trapezius
    e) external intercostals

The Respiratory System

16. a) **FALSE** The lung and pleura extend about 4 cm above the middle of the clavicle on both sides.
    b) **TRUE**
    c) **FALSE** It lies along the fourth costal cartilage.
    d) **TRUE** The upper lobe bronchus is given off outside the lung.
    e) **TRUE** It is separated from it by the diaphragm.

17. a) **TRUE** The principal (primary) bronchus gives off the lobar bronchi which give rise to the segmental bronchi.
    b) **FALSE** It passes posteriorly, and foreign bodies (and aspirated fluid) can enter it when the patient lies on his back.
    c) **FALSE** The finer bronchi are lined by cuboidal epithelium, and the alveoli by very flat cells.
    d) **FALSE** The respiratory bronchioles are finer and more distal; they have alveoli opening from their walls.
    e) **TRUE**

18. a) **FALSE** The lower border of the parietal pleura is about two ribs below that of the lung.
    b) **FALSE** The visceral pleura is innervated by autonomic nerves.
    c) **FALSE** The visceral pleura does; it fits the lung closely.
    d) **TRUE** For about 3–4 cm.
    e) **TRUE** The artery lies on the apex of the lung and pleura.

19. a) **TRUE**
    b) **TRUE**
    c) **TRUE**
    d) **FALSE** Trapezius is not attached to the ribs.
    e) **TRUE**

The Respiratory System

20. **The bronchial arteries**
    a) carry blood to alveoli in the lung
    b) carry oxygen-poor blood to conducting and supporting tissues in the lung
    c) are branches of the pulmonary arteries
    d) are usually branches of the aorta
    e) are normally four in number

21. **A patient is stabbed in the chest, the knife passing posteriorly straight through the anterior extremity of the fifth left intercostal space. The following structures may be injured:**
    a) the left pleural sac
    b) the right pleural sac
    c) the pericardial sac
    d) the superior epigastric artery
    e) the inferior vena cava

22. **When the diaphragm descends in inspiration, the following structures are enlarged:**
    a) the oesophageal hiatus
    b) the aperture for the inferior vena cava
    c) the aperture for the internal thoracic artery
    d) the aortic hiatus
    e) the thoracic duct

23. **Cancer of the apex of the lung may affect certain vital structures which cross the neck of the first rib. This could result in**
    a) paralysis of one hemidiaphragm
    b) loss of sweating from half of the face
    c) impaired opposition of the thumb
    d) inability to close the eyelid completely
    e) loss of cutaneous sensation in the first intercostal space

The Respiratory System

20. a) **FALSE** They supply blood to the lung only as far as the respiratory bronchioles.
    b) **FALSE** They supply oxygen-rich blood to these tissues.
    c) **FALSE**
    d) **TRUE** The right bronchial artery may come from the posterior intercostal artery.
    e) **FALSE** The number varies, but usually there are three.

21. a) **TRUE** The anterior limit of the sac is along the lateral border of the sternum.
    b) **FALSE** The right sac does not extend beyond the middle of the sternum.
    c) **TRUE** As it lies behind the pleural sac.
    d) **FALSE** The superior epigastric artery is usually given off in the sixth intercostal space.
    e) **FALSE** This terminates at the level of the right sixth sternocostal junction.

22. a) **FALSE**
    b) **TRUE**
    c) **FALSE**
    d) **FALSE**
    e) **FALSE**

23. a) **FALSE** The phrenic nerve is not related to the neck of the rib.
    b) **TRUE** Due to paralysis of the sympathetic trunk (stellate ganglion).
    c) **TRUE** Due to paralysis of the first thoracic nerve.
    d) **FALSE** Orbicularis oculi, which closes the eyelid, is supplied by the facial nerve.
    e) **FALSE** This area is supplied by the supraclavicular nerves (C3 and C4).

The Respiratory System

24. With respect to the trachea and bronchi:
   a) the carina is at the level of the suprasternal notch
   b) inhaled safety pins are more apt to enter the right main bronchus
   c) the left bronchus is longer and branches outside the lung
   d) the bifurcation angle is the same in infants and adults
   e) the trachea moves upward with the larynx during swallowing

The Respiratory System

24. a) **FALSE** It is at the level of the angle of the sternum.
 b) **TRUE**
 c) **FALSE** It is longer but all its branches are given off inside the lung.
 d) **FALSE** The angle is wider in infants and the two bronchi slope more or less equally, unlike the case in the adult.
 e) **FALSE** The trachea is elastic; it can stretch.

The Respiratory System

Picture questions

Question 1
1. ___
2. ___
3. ___
4. ___
5. ___
6. ___
7. ___
8. ___
9. ___
10. ___
11. ___
12. ___

A. Frontal sinus
B. Cribriform plate
C. Inferior concha
D. Bony palate
E. Cranial cavity
F. Superior concha
G. Sphenoidal sinus
H. Middle concha
I. Tubal elevation
J. Soft palate
K. Anterior arch of atlas
L. Opening of auditory tube

The Respiratory System

Question 2
1. ___
2. ___
3. ___
4. ___
5. ___
6. ___
7. ___
8. ___
9. ___
10. ___

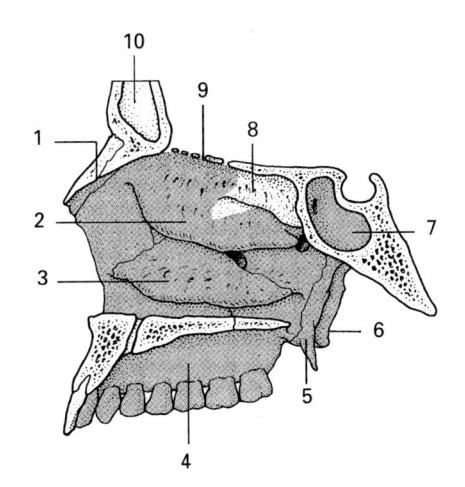

A. Lateral pterygoid plate
B. Medial pterygoid plate
C. Sphenoidal sinus
D. Alveolar process
E. Superior concha
F. Inferior concha
G. Cribriform plate of ethmoid
H. Middle concha
I. Frontal sinus
J. Nasal bone

Question 3
1. ___
2. ___
3. ___
4. ___
5. ___
6. ___
7. ___
8. ___
9. ___
10. ___

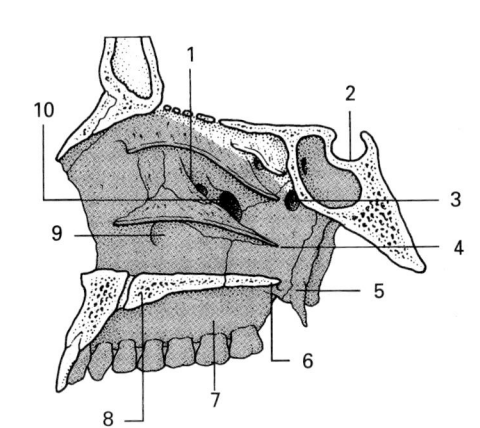

A. Infundibulum
B. Medial pterygoid plate
C. Sphenopalatine foramen
D. Palatal plate of maxilla
E. Hypophyseal fossa
F. Horizontal portion of palatine bone
G. Opening of nasolacrimal duct
H. Vertical portion of palatine bone
I. Opening of maxillary sinus
J. Alveolar process

The Respiratory System

Question 4
1. ____
2. ____
3. ____
4. ____
5. ____
6. ____
7. ____
8. ____
9. ____
10. ____
11. ____
12. ____
13. ____

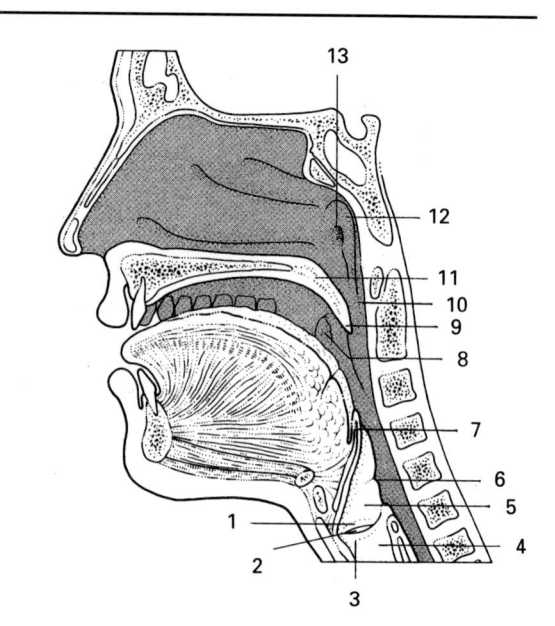

A. Ventricle
B. Pharyngeal isthmus
C. Aryepiglottic fold
D. Vestibular fold
E. Opening of eustachian tube
F. Palatine tonsil
G. Tubal elevation
H. Vocal fold
I. Epiglottis
J. Infraglottic larynx
K. Vestibule
L. Soft palate
M. Uvula

The Respiratory System

Question 5
1. ____
2. ____
3. ____
4. ____
5. ____
6. ____

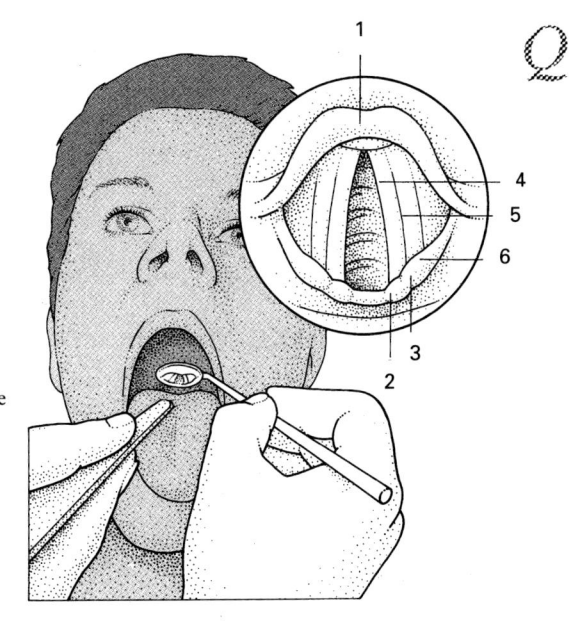

    A. Epiglottis
    B. Cuneiform cartilage
    C. Vestibular fold
    D. Corniculate cartilage
    E. Vocal fold
    F. Aryepiglottic fold

Question 6
1. ____
2. ____
3. ____
4. ____
5. ____
6. ____
7. ____
8. ____
9. ____
10. ____

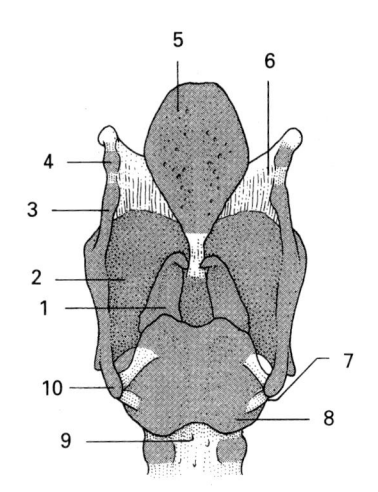

    A. Cricoid cartilage
    B. Superior cornu of thyroid cartilage
    C. Epiglottis
    D. Cricothyroid joint
    E. Cricotracheal ligament
    F. Lamina of thyroid cartilage
    G. Cartilago triticea
    H. Thyrohyoid ligament
    I. Arytenoid cartilage
    J. Inferior cornu of thyroid cartilage

Answers on page 252

The Respiratory System

Question 7
1. ____
2. ____
3. ____
4. ____
5. ____

    A. Cricothyroid joint
    B. Cricoid cartilage
    C. Thyroid notch
    D. Thyroid cartilage
    E. Thyrohyoid ligament

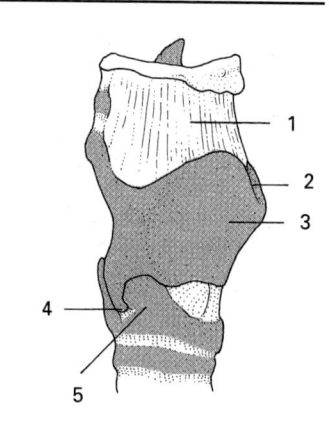

Question 8
1. ____
2. ____
3. ____
4. ____
5. ____

    A. Ventricle
    B. Epiglottis
    C. Quadrangular membrane
    D. Cricovocal membrane
    E. Aryepiglottic fold

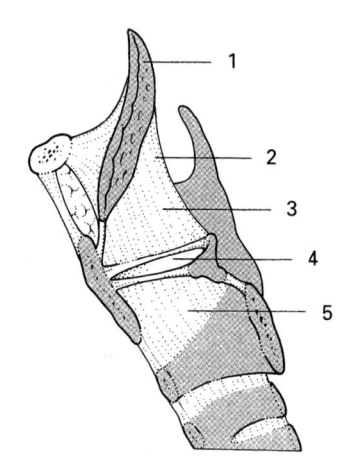

The Respiratory System

Question 9
1. ____
2. ____
3. ____
4. ____
5. ____
6. ____
7. ____
8. ____
9. ____

A. Sternohyoid
B. Internal jugular vein
C. Pharynx
D. Vagus nerve
E. Common carotid artery
F. Thyroid gland
G. Larynx
H. Sternothyroid
I. Carotid sheath

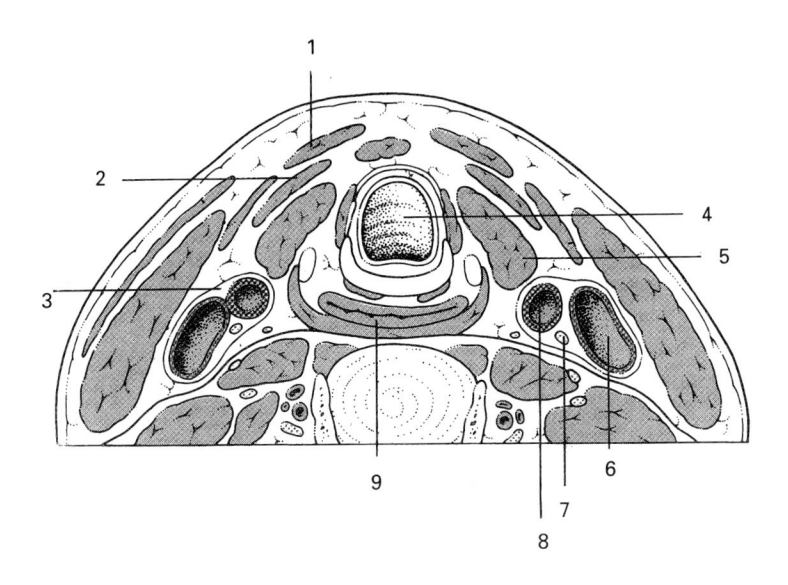

Answers on pages 252 and 253

The Respiratory System

Question 10
1. ____
2. ____
3. ____
4. ____

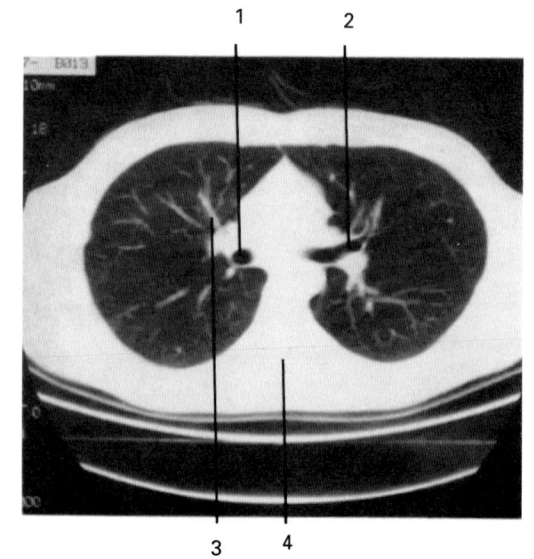

A. Vertebra
B. Right bronchus
C. Lung vessels
D. Left bronchus

The Respiratory System

Question 11

1. ___
2. ___
3. ___
4. ___
5. ___
6. ___
7. ___
8. ___

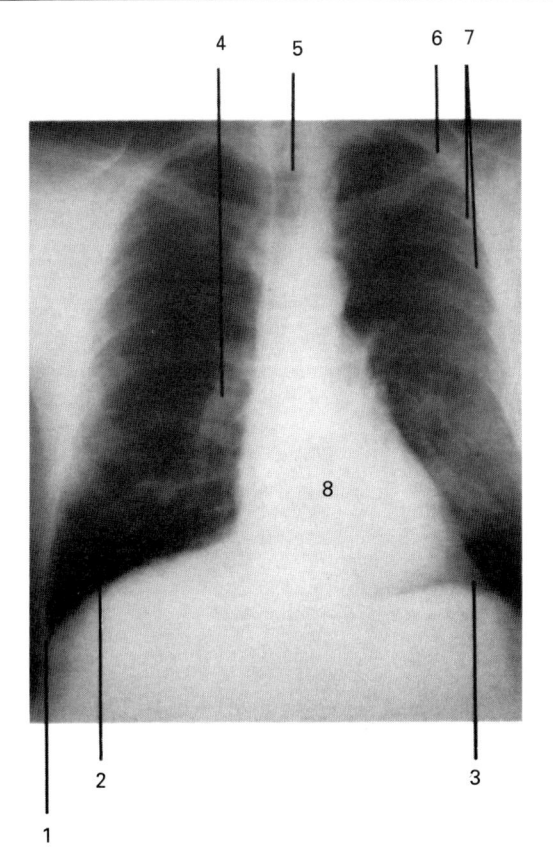

A. Diaphragm
B. Clavicle
C. Heart shadow
D. Costo-diaphragmatic recess
E. Blood vessels in the lung
F. Ribs
G. Trachea
H. Diaphragm

Answers on page 253

The Respiratory System

Question 12

1. ____
2. ____
3. ____
4. ____
5. ____
6. ____
7. ____
8. ____
9. ____
10. ____
11. ____
12. ____
13. ____

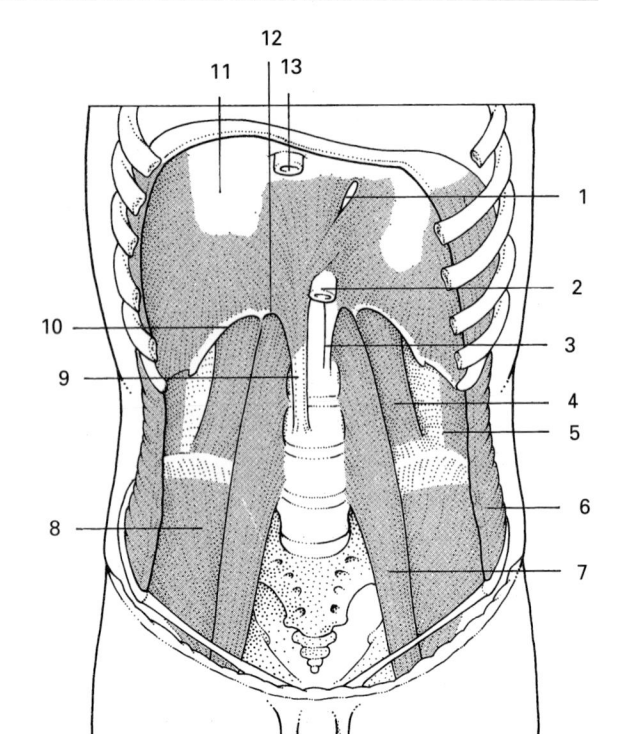

A. Lateral arcuate ligament
B. Left crus of diaphragm
C. Right crus of diaphragm
D. Quadratus lumborum
E. Central tendon of diaphragm
F. Aorta
G. Oesophageal orifice
H. Medial arcuate ligament
I. Iliacus
J. Psoas major
K. Transversus abdominis
L. Inferior vena cava
M. External oblique abdominis

250

The Respiratory System

Picture questions *A*

Question 1
1. **A** Frontal sinus
2. **B** Cribriform plate
3. **F** Superior concha
4. **H** Middle concha
5. **C** Inferior concha
6. **I** Tubal elevation
7. **D** Bony palate
8. **K** Anterior arch of atlas
9. **J** Soft palate
10. **L** Opening of auditory tube
11. **E** Cranial cavity
12. **G** Sphenoidal sinus

Question 2
1. **J** Nasal bone
2. **H** Middle concha
3. **F** Inferior concha
4. **D** Alveolar process
5. **B** Medial pterygoid plate
6. **A** Lateral pterygoid plate
7. **C** Sphenoidal sinus
8. **E** Superior concha
9. **G** Cribriform plate of ethmoid
10. **I** Frontal sinus

Question 3
1. **A** Infundibulum
2. **E** Hypophyseal fossa
3. **C** Sphenopalatine foramen
4. **H** Vertical portion of palatine bone
5. **B** Medial pterygoid plate
6. **F** Horizontal portion of palatine bone
7. **J** Alveolar process
8. **D** Palatal plate of maxilla
9. **G** Opening of nasolacrimal duct
10. **I** Opening of maxillary sinus

The Respiratory System

A Question 4
1. **D** Vestibular fold
2. **A** Ventricle
3. **H** Vocal fold
4. **J** Infraglottic larynx
5. **K** Vestibule
6. **C** Aryepiglottic fold
7. **I** Epiglottis
8. **F** Palatine tonsil
9. **M** Uvula
10. **B** Pharyngeal isthmus
11. **L** Soft palate
12. **G** Tubal elevation
13. **E** Opening of eustachian tube

Question 5
1. **A** Epiglottis
2. **D** Corniculate cartilage
3. **B** Cuneiform cartilage
4. **E** Vocal fold
5. **C** Vestibular fold
6. **F** Aryepiglottic fold

Question 6
1. **I** Arytenoid cartilage
2. **F** Lamina of thyroid cartilage
3. **B** Superior cornu of thyroid cartilage
4. **G** Cartilago triticea
5. **C** Epiglottis
6. **H** Thyrohyoid ligament
7. **D** Cricothyroid joint
8. **A** Cricoid cartilage
9. **E** Cricotracheal ligament
10. **J** Inferior cornu of thyroid cartilage

Question 7
1. **E** Thyrohyoid ligament
2. **C** Thyroid notch
3. **D** Thyroid cartilage
4. **A** Cricothyroid joint
5. **B** Cricoid cartilage

The Respiratory System

Question 8
1. **B** Epiglottis
2. **E** Aryepiglottic fold
3. **C** Quadrangular membrane
4. **A** Ventricle
5. **D** Cricovocal membrane

Question 9
1. **A** Sternohyoid
2. **H** Sternothyroid
3. **I** Carotid sheath
4. **G** Larynx
5. **F** Thyroid gland
6. **B** Internal jugular vein
7. **D** Vagus nerve
8. **E** Common carotid artery
9. **C** Pharynx

Question 10
1. **B** Right bronchus
2. **D** Left bronchus
3. **C** Lung vessels
4. **A** Vertebra

Question 11
1. **D** Costodiaphragmatic recess
2. **A** Diaphragm
3. **H** Diaphragm
4. **E** Blood vessels in the lung
5. **G** Trachea
6. **B** Clavicle
7. **F** Ribs
8. **C** Heart shadow

The Respiratory System

A Question 12
1. **G** Oesophageal orifice
2. **F** Aorta
3. **B** Left crus of diaphragm
4. **D** Quadratus lumborum
5. **K** Transversus abdominis
6. **M** External oblique abdominis
7. **J** Psoas major
8. **I** Iliacus
9. **C** Right crus of diaphragm
10. **A** Lateral arcuate ligament
11. **E** Central tendon of diaphragm
12. **H** Medial arcuate ligament
13. **L** Inferior vena cava

The Respiratory System

Clinical problems

1. Bleeding from the nasal cavity (epistaxis) is a common condition and may be due to a variety of causes including nose picking (epistaxis digitorum). What may be the source of the bleeding? What immediate treatment is advocated when faced with a nose bleed? In severe cases ligation of arteries is advised. Will ligation of the external carotid artery alone always stop epistaxis?

2. Why is infection of the paranasal sinuses (sinusitis) common? How may infection spread from one sinus to another? Where might one feel the pain in infection of the maxima and frontal sinuses? Why is maxillary sinusitis difficult to clear?

3. Conditions producing obstruction of the upper respiratory air passage may require a tracheostomy to make the patient breathe. Such conditions include acute infections of the epiglottis and larynx, especially in children, foreign body impaction and tumour of the larynx. In this operation the second, third and often the fourth tracheal rings are divided to insert a tracheostomy tube. What structure will the surgeon come across while exposing the tracheal rings? Why is it not usually performed at a higher level? Why is this operation more difficult in a child? In a dire emergency an opening made in the cricothyroid ligament may be life saving. Will this opening be above or below the level of the vocal cords?

Answers on page 256 255

The Respiratory System

A Clinical problems

1. Bleeding from the nose may be arterial or venous. In about 90% of cases it may be from the Littles' area in the anterior part of the septum where most of the vessels anastomose. The nasal cavity is supplied by the sphenopalatine branch of the maxillary, septal branch of the facial as well as the anterior and posterior ethmoidal branches from the ophthalmic (internal carotid). The immediate treatment is to make the person sit up and apply pressure to the nose by pinching it for about 10 minutes. If this does not stop the bleeding nasal 'packs' may be inserted after anaesthetising the mucosa with a local spray. Ligation of the external carotid alone may not be sufficient to stop the bleeding as the ethmoidal branches are from the ophthalmic division of the internal carotid artery.

2. Sinusitis usually occurs as an extension of infection from the nasal cavity. It can also extend from an infected tooth to which the maxillary sinus is related. The frontal, maxillary and ethmoidal sinuses open into the middle meatus of the nasal cavity very close to each other and when one sinus is affected the infection can easily spread to another. The maxillary sinus opening is in the upper part of its medial wall and hence not in the most dependent position. Drainage is difficult when infected. The maxillary sinus is supplied by the infraorbital nerve and the pain and tenderness in sinusitis are present in the region over the maxilla on the face. Sometimes the pain may be referred along the branches of the infraorbital nerve and manifest as toothache.

3. While performing a classical tracheostomy the surgeon will come across skin, superficial fascia, the anterior jugular vein, the investing layer of fascia, the infrahyoid muscles and the isthmus of the thyroid gland in front of the second, third and fourth tracheal rings. Removal of the first ring often results in laryngeal stenosis. In an infant the trachea is much narrower, the neck is shorter and the major vessels such as the brachiocephalic veins may be lying in front of the cervical part of the trachea. An opening made into the cricothyroid ligament will be below the level of the vocal cords.

The Respiratory System

4. A flexible fibreoptic bronchoscope can be introduced into the trachea and advanced into the bronchi for examination of the airway. Which nerves of the larynx and trachea are anaesthetised to facilitate this examination? Arterial pulsation may be visible on the tracheal wall. Which artery produces the pulsation? The carina is seen at the bifurcation of the trachea. What is its normal appearance? It is easier to advance the tube down the right main bronchus. Why? Openings of how many lobar bronchi will be seen on the right side? Openings of the segmental bronchi may also be visualised. What is a segmental bronchus? Which is the first segmental bronchus seen going in a posterior direction?

5. Knowledge of the surface anatomy of the respiratory system is important in physical examination of the chest. Where does one feel the trachea? What is the lower limit of the pleural cavity and that of the lung? What is the relation of the pleural cavity to the clavicle and the sternum? Which ribs mark the levels of the oblique and horizontal fissures?

The Respiratory System

4. The sensory innervation of the larynx is through the internal laryngeal and the recurrent laryngeal nerves. The latter supply the part of the larynx below the vocal cords and the trachea. The pulsation seen on the trachea will be that of the arch of the aorta which lies on the wall of the trachea on the left side. The carina is seen as a sharp, shining vertical ridge. It is easier to advance the scope to the right side as the right bronchus is more vertical, hence more in line with the trachea and it is also wider. The right bronchus gives rise to three lobar bronchi. The segmental bronchi are branches of the lobar bronchi. The apical branch of the lower lobe bronchus is the first posterior branch.

5. The trachea is a midline structure and is felt in the lower part of the neck between the two sternocleidomastoid muscles. The pleural cavity extends downwards to a line connecting the 6th rib in front, 8th rib in the midclavicular line, 10th rib in the mid-axillary line and 12th rib at the back. The lower border of the lung is about two ribs above that of the pleura. The lung and pleura extend for about 3 cm above the medial part of the clavicle. Behind the body of the sternum the right pleural cavity lies in the midline and the left starts in the midline and deviates to the lateral border. Behind the manubrium both the pleural cavities deviate toward the sternoclavicular joint. The 6th rib marks the oblique fissure and the right 4th rib the horizontal fissure.

The Cardiovascular System

The Cardiovascular System

THE HEART AND GREAT VESSELS

True/False

1. **The left border of the 'cardiac shadow' in a chest X-ray AP view includes**
   a) the right pulmonary artery
   b) the left atrium
   c) the left ventricle
   d) the aortic arch ('knuckle' or 'knob')
   e) the pulmonary trunk

2. **A stab wound that nicks the anterior surface of the heart could injure**
   a) the great cardiac vein
   b) the coronary sinus
   c) the atrioventricular node
   d) the left atrium
   e) the mitral valve

3. **With respect to the heart:**
   a) the function of the papillary muscles is to open the atrioventricular valves
   b) the left coronary artery supplies the greater part of the left ventricular wall
   c) contraction of the atria is primarily responsible for filling the ventricles
   d) the base of the heart rests on the diaphragm
   e) the apex is at the junction of the two ventricles

The Cardiovascular System

THE HEART AND GREAT VESSELS

1. a) **FALSE** It includes the pulmonary trunk.
   b) **FALSE** The left atrium is a posterior chamber but the left auricle contributes to the left border.
   c) **TRUE** It forms the major portion.
   d) **TRUE** Above the left auricle.
   e) **TRUE** Below the aortic knuckle.

2. a) **TRUE** It lies in the anterior interventricular groove.
   b) **FALSE** It is posterior.
   c) **FALSE** It lies not on the surface but in the interatrial septum above the opening of the coronary sinus.
   d) **FALSE** This chamber is posterior.
   e) **FALSE** It is placed more posteriorly.

3. a) **FALSE** They act to prevent the atrioventricular valves from prolapsing into the atrium in systole.
   b) **TRUE** And part of the anterior wall of the right ventricle.
   c) **FALSE** Most of the ventricular filling is due to the pressure gradient generated by ventricular diastole.
   d) **FALSE** The base of the heart is the left atrium. It faces the oesophagus posteriorly.
   e) **FALSE** The apex is formed entirely by the left ventricle.

The Cardiovascular System

4. **With respect to the innervation of the heart:**
   a) all sympathetic innervation is from the thoracic sympathetic ganglia
   b) the sinoatrial node is supplied by the left vagus nerve
   c) the right vagus nerve supplies the right lung but not the heart
   d) part of the sympathetic innervation of the heart is via the greater splanchnic nerve
   e) the atrioventricular node is supplied by the right vagus nerve

5. **The sinoatrial node**
   a) is located in the wall of the right atrium
   b) lies near the crista terminalis
   c) lies near the inferior vena cava
   d) always receives its blood supply from the right coronary artery
   e) is connected to the AV node by Purkinje fibres

6. **The right atrium**
   a) is completely derived from the right horn of the sinus venosus
   b) is mostly supplied by the left coronary artery
   c) has musculi pectinati on its wall
   d) has valves at the orifices of the superior and inferior venae cavae
   e) has the AV node in the interatrial septum

7. **The right coronary artery**
   a) arises from the arch of the aorta
   b) usually supplies the whole of the right ventricle
   c) usually supplies the atrioventricular node
   d) gives off a posterior interventricular branch
   e) is accompanied by the anterior cardiac veins

The Cardiovascular System

4. a) **FALSE** The three cervical sympathetic ganglia each give off cardiac nerves.
   b) **TRUE** The left and right vagus nerves and their recurrent laryngeal branches give off cardiac branches.
   c) **FALSE**
   d) **FALSE** The splanchnic nerves supply the abdominal viscera.
   e) **TRUE** Through the cardiac plexus.

5. a) **TRUE**
   b) **TRUE** Where the crista meets the superior vena cava.
   c) **FALSE** It lies near the superior vena cava.
   d) **FALSE** This is true only in about 60% of cases; the rest through the left coronary.
   e) **FALSE** There are no Purkinje fibres in the atria.

6. a) **FALSE** It also derives in part from the primitive atrium.
   b) **FALSE** It is mostly supplied by the right coronary artery.
   c) **TRUE** This part is derived from the primitive atrium.
   d) **FALSE** The IVC has a ridge which is the remains of the fetal valve.
   e) **TRUE** Just above the opening of the coronary sinus.

7. a) **FALSE** The right coronary artery originates from the right (anterior) aortic sinus on the ascending aorta.
   b) **FALSE** Part of the anterior surface of the right ventricle is supplied by branches of the anterior interventricular (descending) artery from the left coronary artery.
   c) **TRUE** In 90% of cases, the posterior interventricular artery which supplies the AV node is a branch of the right coronary artery.
   d) **TRUE** The bundle of His is supplied by the posterior interventricular artery.
   e) **FALSE** These veins drain directly into the right atrium.

The Cardiovascular System

Q 8. **The left coronary artery**
   a) lies between the pulmonary trunk and the left auricle ___
   b) arises from the left aortic sinus ___
   c) gives off an anterior interventricular branch ___
   d) has no anastomoses with the right coronary artery ___
   e) often supplies the AV node ___

9. **The anterior interventricular (descending) branch of the left coronary artery**
   a) supplies most of the interventricular septum ___
   b) gives off the left marginal artery ___
   c) continues onto the diaphragmatic surface of the heart ___
   d) generally anastomoses with the posterior interventricular branch of the right coronary artery ___
   e) gives off the diagonal arteries ___

10. **The blood supply from the myocardium returns to the right atrium via**
    a) the coronary sinus ___
    b) the venae cordis minimae ___
    c) the anterior cardiac veins ___
    d) the oblique vein of the left atrium ___
    e) the great cardiac vein ___

11. **The pericardium**
    a) is attached to the sternum ___
    b) has an oblique sinus between the left atrium and the oesophagus ___
    c) is innervated by the phrenic nerve ___
    d) develops from the septum transversum ___
    e) is adherent to the central tendon of the diaphragm ___

The Cardiovascular System

8. a) **TRUE** The stem of the artery lies here as it comes forward from its origin.
   b) **TRUE** It is also known as the left posterior aortic sinus.
   c) **TRUE** This anastomoses with the posterior interventricular branch on the inferior surface of the heart.
   d) **FALSE** But the anastomoses may not be sufficient to prevent an infarction if a major branch is blocked.
   e) **FALSE** In 90% of people the AV node is supplied by the right coronary artery.

9. a) **TRUE** It supplies about two-thirds of the septum.
   b) **TRUE** The latter is often known as the obtuse marginal artery.
   c) **TRUE** To anastomose with the posterior interventricular artery.
   d) **TRUE** The anastomosis is on the diaphragmatic surface.
   e) **TRUE** To supply the left ventricle.

10. a) **TRUE** Most of the cardiac veins are its tributaries.
    b) **TRUE** These are small veins draining directly into the chambers of the heart.
    c) **TRUE** These drain directly into the right atrium.
    d) **TRUE** This vein joins the coronary sinus.
    e) **TRUE** This also joins the coronary sinus.

11. a) **TRUE** They are connected by weak sternopericardial ligaments.
    b) **TRUE** This is part of the pericardial cavity and allows expansion of the left atrium.
    c) **TRUE** The fibrous pericardium is innervated by the phrenic nerve.
    d) **TRUE** The fibrous pericardium is derived from the septum transversum.
    e) **TRUE** Because the central tendon also develops from the septum transversum.

The Cardiovascular System

12. **The pericardial sac may be aspirated without entering the pleural cavity**
    a) immediately to the right of the sternum through the sixth intercostal space
    b) immediately to the left of the sternum through the fourth intercostal space
    c) 2.5 cm to either side of the sternum in the third intercostal space
    d) between the xiphoid and the left eighth costal cartilage through the central tendon
    e) through the fifth intercostal space in the midclavicular line on the left side

13. **The arch of the aorta**
    a) begins opposite the left third costal cartilage at its junction with the sternum
    b) extends superiorly to the suprasternal notch
    c) gives off the coronary arteries
    d) gives off the left subclavian artery
    e) gives off the right subclavian artery

14. **The arch of the aorta**
    a) is crossed on its left side by the left phrenic nerve
    b) lies almost in a sagittal plane
    c) lies on the left surface of the trachea
    d) usually causes an impression on the oesophagus
    e) is closely related to the right recurrent laryngeal nerve

15. **The arch of the aorta**
    a) lies partly in the pericardial cavity
    b) lies totally in the superior mediastinum
    c) normally has three branches
    d) is directly in contact with the right and left vagus nerves
    e) has the ligamentum arteriosum attached to its inferior surface

The Cardiovascular System

12. a) **FALSE** This is almost the lower limit of the heart and pericardium.
    b) **TRUE** This occasionally produces pneumothorax.
    c) **FALSE** This will produce pneumothorax.
    d) **TRUE** This is usually the preferred route.
    e) **FALSE** The apex of the heart usually lies medial to this point.

13. a) **FALSE** It begins as a continuation of the ascending aorta behind the sternum at the level of the second costal cartilage.
    b) **FALSE** In the adult, it extends halfway up the manubrium sterni. In infants it extends higher.
    c) **FALSE** These arise from the ascending aorta.
    d) **TRUE** And also the left common carotid.
    e) **FALSE** This is not a direct branch but is given off by the brachiocephalic trunk from the arch of the aorta.

14. a) **TRUE** It is also crossed by the left vagus and the left superior intercostal vein.
    b) **TRUE** It passes backwards over the left bronchus to reach the body of the T4 vertebra.
    c) **TRUE** The arch of the aorta separates the left lung from the trachea. Also, aortic pulsations are visible when the interior of the trachea is examined in the living.
    d) **TRUE** This may cause difficulty in swallowing when there is an aneurysm of the arch of the aorta.
    e) **FALSE** The left nerve winds round the ligamentum arteriosum and the arch of the aorta.

15. a) **FALSE** The ascending aorta lies partly in the pericardial cavity.
    b) **TRUE** At the lower border of the T4 vertebra, it becomes the descending aorta.
    c) **TRUE** They are the brachiocephalic trunk, the left common carotid and the left subclavian.
    d) **FALSE** Only with the left vagus. The right vagus lies on the surface of the trachea.
    e) **TRUE** This extends from the commencement of the left pulmonary artery.

The Cardiovascular System

16. **The pulmonary trunk**
    a) is intrapericardial
    b) shares a pericardial sleeve with the ascending aorta
    c) is separated from the left atrium by the oblique (pericardial) sinus
    d) develops from the truncus arteriosus
    e) divides into the left and right pulmonary arteries

17. **The ductus arteriosus joins the aorta and**
    a) the pulmonary vein
    b) the left pulmonary artery
    c) the bronchial vein
    d) the coronary sinus
    e) the right pulmonary artery

18. **The ductus arteriosus**
    a) is closely related to the phrenic nerve
    b) in the fetus shunts blood from the aorta to the pulmonary artery
    c) is closely related to the left recurrent laryngeal nerve
    d) when patent after birth shunts blood from the aorta to the pulmonary artery
    e) is derived from the left sixth aortic arch

19. **The brachiocephalic trunk (artery)**
    a) is the largest of the branches of the aortic arch
    b) gives off its terminal branches behind the right sternoclavicular joint
    c) occasionally gives off the thyroidea ima artery
    d) gives off the right vertebral artery
    e) lies on the right surface of the trachea

The Cardiovascular System

16. a) **TRUE**
   b) **TRUE**
   c) **FALSE** It is separated from the left atrium by the transverse sinus which lies behind the ascending aorta and the pulmonary trunk.
   d) **TRUE** Along with the ascending aorta.
   e) **TRUE**

17. a) **FALSE**
   b) **TRUE**
   c) **FALSE**
   d) **FALSE**
   e) **FALSE**

18. a) **FALSE**
   b) **FALSE** Blood is shunted from the pulmonary artery to the aorta.
   c) **TRUE** The nerve branches off from the vagus at this level.
   d) **TRUE** After birth, the pressure gradient reverses. Aortic pressure becomes greater than that of the pulmonary artery.
   e) **TRUE** The corresponding arch on the right side disappears.

19. a) **TRUE**
   b) **TRUE** They are the right common carotid and the right subclavian arteries.
   c) **TRUE** It may also arise from the arch of the aorta.
   d) **FALSE** This is a branch of the subclavian artery.
   e) **TRUE**

The Cardiovascular System

20. **Branches of the subclavian artery anastomose with branches of**
    a) the external carotid artery
    b) the internal carotid artery
    c) the axillary artery
    d) the descending aorta
    e) the external iliac artery

21. **The right subclavian artery**
    a) is separated by scalenus anterior from the right subclavian vein
    b) is crossed behind by the right vagus nerve
    c) is closely related to the upper trunk of the brachial plexus
    d) is covered by the suprapleural membrane
    e) pulsation can be felt by palpating it against the first rib

22. **The common carotid artery**
    a) is contained inside the carotid sheath
    b) is lateral to the internal jugular vein
    c) is closely related to the sympathetic trunk
    d) has no side branches
    e) terminates at the upper border of the thyroid cartilage

23. **The following statements about the external carotid artery are true:**
    a) the superficial temporal and the maxillary arteries are the terminal branches
    b) it lies external to the internal carotid at its origin
    c) the hypoglossal nerve is a deep relation
    d) the superior laryngeal nerve lies deep to the artery
    e) the glossopharyngeal nerve lies between the external and internal carotid arteries

The Cardiovascular System

20. a) **TRUE**   The inferior thyroid artery (thyrocervical trunk of the subclavian) and superior thyroid artery (external carotid).
    b) **TRUE**   The posterior cerebral artery (basilar, vertebral) and internal carotid in the circle of Willis.
    c) **TRUE**   The suprascapular artery (thyrocervical trunk of subclavian) and subscapular artery (axillary).
    d) **TRUE**   The anterior intercostal arteries (internal mammary) and posterior intercostal arteries (descending aorta).
    e) **TRUE**   The superior epigastric artery (internal mammary) and inferior epigastric artery (external iliac).

21. a) **TRUE**
    b) **FALSE**   It is crossed in front by the vagus nerve.
    c) **FALSE**   It is closely related to the lower trunk of the brachial plexus.
    d) **FALSE**   It lies on the suprapleural membrane.
    e) **TRUE**   At the angle between the lateral border of the sternocleidomastoid and the clavicle.

22. a) **TRUE**   The carotid sheath also contains the internal jugular vein and the vagus nerve.
    b) **FALSE**   The vein is always lateral to the artery, with the vagus nerve between the two.
    c) **TRUE**   It lies behind the carotid sheath.
    d) **TRUE**
    e) **TRUE**   The external and internal carotids are usually given off at this level, but sometimes the division is higher.

23. a) **TRUE**   Its other branches are the superior thyroid, lingual, facial, occipital, posterior auricular and ascending pharyngeal arteries.
    b) **FALSE**   It lies deep to the internal carotid at its origin, but as it ascends becomes more superficial.
    c) **FALSE**   The nerve crosses superficial to the internal and external carotid arteries.
    d) **TRUE**   The nerve lies deep to both carotids.
    e) **TRUE**   The glossopharyngeal nerve accompanies the stylopharyngeus muscle.

The Cardiovascular System

Q

24. **The thoracic aorta (descending aorta)**
    a) lies on the vertebral column throughout its course _____
    b) is crossed behind by the oesophagus _____
    c) pierces the central tendon of the diaphragm _____
    d) gives off nine pairs of posterior intercostal arteries _____
    e) lies on the right side of the oesophagus in its lower part _____

25. **Concerning the common iliac arteries:**
    a) they originate to the left of the midline _____
    b) the ureter crosses posterior to the termination of the artery _____
    c) the iliolumbar artery is a branch _____
    d) the common iliac veins are posterior relations _____
    e) the inferior mesenteric vessels cross in front of the left common iliac artery _____

26. **Branches of the internal iliac artery include**
    a) the uterine artery _____
    b) the superior gluteal artery _____
    c) the superior rectal artery _____
    d) the inferior gluteal artery _____
    e) the inferior epigastric artery _____

27. **The superior vena cava**
    a) is entirely extrapericardial _____
    b) lies anterior to the transverse sinus _____
    c) has the right vagus on its lateral surface _____
    d) receives the azygos vein _____
    e) is formed at the level of the second right costal cartilage _____

The Cardiovascular System

24. a) **TRUE** Between the T4–T12 vertebrae.
    b) **FALSE** The oesophagus crosses in front of the aorta.
    c) **FALSE** It passes between the two crura.
    d) **TRUE**
    e) **TRUE** The aorta is in the midline, the oesophagus is to the left.

25. a) **TRUE** By bifurcation of the aorta.
    b) **FALSE** It crosses anterior.
    c) **FALSE** It is a branch of the internal iliac artery.
    d) **TRUE** At this level, the veins are posterior to the arteries.
    e) **TRUE**

26. a) **TRUE**
    b) **TRUE**
    c) **FALSE** This is a continuation of the inferior mesenteric artery.
    d) **TRUE**
    e) **FALSE** This is derived from the external iliac artery.

27. a) **FALSE** The lower part is surrounded by pericardium.
    b) **FALSE** The transverse sinus is anterior.
    c) **FALSE** The right phrenic nerve is on its lateral surface.
    d) **TRUE** At the level of the right 2nd costal cartilage.
    e) **FALSE** It is formed at the lower border of the first right costal cartilage by the union of the two brachiocephalic veins.

The Cardiovascular System

28. **The brachiocephalic veins**
    a) are formed by the union of the internal jugular and subclavian veins
    b) are formed behind the right and left sternoclavicular joints respectively
    c) are furnished with valves
    d) open directly into the right atrium
    e) are related to the right and left phrenic nerves respectively

29. **The left brachiocephalic vein**
    a) is formed by the union of the internal jugular and subclavian veins
    b) lies behind the upper half of the manubrium sterni
    c) receives the inferior thyroid veins
    d) receives the left vertebral vein
    e) receives the left superior intercostal vein

30. **Regarding the internal jugular vein:**
    a) it commences as a continuation of the sigmoid sinus
    b) it lies medial to the carotid arteries
    c) blood may be aspirated from the vein by inserting a needle between the sternal and the clavicular heads of the sternocleidomastoid
    d) the inferior thyroid veins are tributaries
    e) it is closely associated with lymph nodes

31. **The inferior vena cava**
    a) is formed at the level of the fourth lumbar vertebra
    b) pierces the right crus of the diaphragm at the level of the twelfth thoracic vertebra
    c) has the inferior mesenteric vein as a tributary
    d) is joined by the testicular veins
    e) lies to the right of the abdominal aorta

The Cardiovascular System

28. a) **TRUE**
    b) **TRUE**
    c) **FALSE** The brachiocephalic veins, the superior vena cava and the common iliac veins are all devoid of valves.
    d) **FALSE** They join together to form the superior vena cava.
    e) **FALSE** The right nerve lies on the lateral surface of the right vein.

29. a) **TRUE**
    b) **TRUE** It crosses behind the sternum obliquely from left to right.
    c) **TRUE**
    d) **TRUE** It receives the right vertebral vein as well.
    e) **TRUE**

30. a) **TRUE** Just below the jugular foramen.
    b) **FALSE** The vein lies lateral to both the internal and the common carotid arteries.
    c) **TRUE** But if the needle is advanced further it may puncture the pleura and the lung.
    d) **FALSE** Its tributaries are the superior and middle thyroid veins, along with the lingual, facial and pharyngeal veins.
    e) **TRUE** The deep cervical lymph nodes lie on the vein and may become adherent to it if involved in malignancy or inflammation.

31. a) **FALSE** It starts at the level of the L5 vertebra.
    b) **FALSE** It pierces the central tendon at the level of T8.
    c) **FALSE** This drains into the splenic vein and then into the portal system.
    d) **FALSE** Only the right testicular vein joins the inferior vena cava; the left vein joins the left renal vein.
    e) **TRUE**

The Cardiovascular System

32. The external iliac vein
  a) is lateral to the external iliac artery at its commencement ____
  b) is a continuation of the femoral vein ____
  c) joins the internal iliac vein anterior to the sacroiliac joint ____
  d) is crossed by the ductus deferens in the male ____
  e) is joined by the fifth lumbar vein ____

The Cardiovascular System

32. a) **FALSE** The vein is medial.
   b) **TRUE**
   c) **TRUE**
   d) **TRUE** The ductus crosses the external iliac artery and vein.
   e) **FALSE** This usually joins the iliolumbar vein.

The Cardiovascular System

THE BLOOD SUPPLY OF THE TRUNK AND LIMBS
True/False

33. **The internal thoracic artery, which is often used to bypass a blocked coronary artery**
    a) is a branch of the axillary artery
    b) has no terminal branches
    c) descends posterior to the sternum
    d) supplies the mammary gland
    e) has branches that anastomose with those of the descending aorta

34. **The inferior epigastric artery**
    a) originates from the internal iliac
    b) lies lateral to the deep inguinal ring
    c) anastomoses with the superior epigastric artery
    d) lies in the rectus sheath
    e) may enlarge in coarctation of the aorta

35. **The azygos vein**
    a) drains into the right brachiocephalic vein
    b) passes through the diaphragm at the level of the tenth thoracic vertebra
    c) is connected to the vertebral venous plexuses
    d) is closely related to the upper lobe of the right lung
    e) will enlarge in inferior vena caval obstructions

36. **The superior mesenteric artery**
    a) arises from the abdominal aorta in front of the neck of the pancreas
    b) gives off the inferior pancreaticoduodenal artery
    c) supplies the left colic flexure
    d) may occasionally give off the hepatic artery
    e) lies at the root of the mesentery

The Cardiovascular System

THE BLOOD SUPPLY OF THE TRUNK AND LIMBS A

33. a) **FALSE** It is a branch of the subclavian artery.
    b) **FALSE** It terminates by dividing into the superior epigastric and musculophrenic arteries.
    c) **FALSE** It descends one finger's breadth lateral to the sternum.
    d) **TRUE**
    e) **TRUE** The anterior intercostal arteries from the internal mammary, and the posterior intercostal arteries from the aorta anastomose in the intercostal spaces.

34. a) **FALSE** It is a branch of the external iliac artery.
    b) **FALSE** It lies medial to the deep ring.
    c) **TRUE**
    d) **TRUE**
    e) **TRUE**

35. a) **FALSE** It joins the superior vena cava.
    b) **FALSE** It passes through the aortic orifice at the level of T12.
    c) **TRUE**
    d) **TRUE** It may deeply indent the lobe, producing the azygos lobe.
    e) **TRUE** As it connects the two venae cavae.

36. a) **FALSE** It arises behind the neck of the pancreas.
    b) **TRUE**
    c) **FALSE** It usually anastomoses with branches of the inferior mesenteric artery to the right of the left colic flexure.
    d) **TRUE**
    e) **TRUE**

The Cardiovascular System

37. **The portal vein**
   a) contains many valves
   b) is constituted by the splenic and superior mesenteric veins
   c) lies in front of the neck of the pancreas
   d) lies behind the first part of the duodenum
   e) drains all the gastrointestinal tract and the suprarenal glands

38. **The portosystemic anastomoses are between**
   a) oesophageal branches of the left gastric and the azygos veins
   b) the superior and inferior mesenteric veins
   c) the superior and inferior epigastric veins
   d) the superior rectal and lumbar veins
   e) the superior and inferior rectal veins

39. **The internal pudendal artery**
   a) leaves the pelvis via the greater sciatic foramen
   b) leaves the pelvis via the lesser sciatic foramen
   c) gives origin to the scrotal arteries
   d) gives origin to the middle rectal artery
   e) lies on the lateral wall of the ischiorectal fossa

40. **The uterine artery**
   a) is a branch of the internal iliac artery
   b) crosses below the ureter near the cervix
   c) supplies the vagina
   d) supplies the uterine tube
   e) does not anastomose with any other artery

The Cardiovascular System

37. a) **FALSE** The portal veins and its tributaries have no valves.
    b) **TRUE** The inferior mesenteric often joins the splenic vein, and sometimes the superior mesenteric.
    c) **FALSE** It lies behind the neck.
    d) **TRUE** Along with the gastroduodenal artery and the bile duct.
    e) **FALSE** The suprarenal veins drain into systemic veins, the left to the renal vein, and the right to the inferior vena cava.

38. a) **TRUE** In the lower part of the oesophagus.
    b) **FALSE** Both veins are components of the portal system.
    c) **FALSE** They are systemic veins.
    d) **FALSE** They do not anastomose.
    e) **TRUE**

39. a) **TRUE** Accompanied by the pudendal nerve.
    b) **FALSE** It enters the perineum through the lesser sciatic foramen.
    c) **TRUE** And the corresponding labial arteries in the female.
    d) **FALSE** This is usually a branch of the internal iliac.
    e) **TRUE** Along with the pudendal nerve.

40. a) **TRUE**
    b) **FALSE** The artery crosses above the ureter.
    c) **TRUE** Many arteries supply the vagina.
    d) **TRUE** This is also supplied by the ovarian artery.
    e) **FALSE** It anastomoses with the ovarian and vaginal arteries.

The Cardiovascular System

41. The axillary artery
   a) begins at the upper border of the clavicle
   b) terminates as it crosses the inferior border of teres minor
   c) is contained in the axillary sheath
   d) has the median nerve anterior to its proximal third
   e) has the radial nerve posterior to its distal third

42. The brachial artery:
   a) is crossed in front by the median nerve in the middle of the arm
   b) lies medial to the median nerve in the cubital fossa
   c) gives off the profunda brachii artery just above teres major
   d) pulsation can be felt lateral to the tendon of biceps in the cubital fossa
   e) sometimes divides above the cubital fossa

43. The cephalic vein
   a) is superficial for most of its course
   b) often lies in the anatomical snuffbox
   c) often lies on the lateral aspect of the lower end of the radius
   d) lies medial to the biceps tendon
   e) may enlarge if the axillary vein is obstructed

44. The femoral artery:
   a) continues as the popliteal artery
   b) gives off the profunda femoris artery
   c) is continuous with the external iliac artery
   d) is lateral to the femoral vein throughout
   e) pulsation can be felt at the midinguinal point

The Cardiovascular System

41. a) **FALSE** It begins at the outer border of the first rib.
    b) **FALSE** It terminates as it crosses the inferior border of teres major.
    c) **TRUE** Along with the components of the brachial plexus.
    d) **FALSE** The nerve is anterior to the distal third.
    e) **TRUE**

42. a) **TRUE** The nerve crosses from lateral to medial.
    b) **FALSE** The nerve is medial.
    c) **FALSE** The profunda brachii is given off below teres major.
    d) **FALSE** The artery lies medial to the tendon of biceps in the cubital fossa.
    e) **TRUE**

43. a) **TRUE** It pierces the clavipectoral fascia.
    b) **TRUE**
    c) **TRUE**
    d) **FALSE** It lies lateral to biceps at the elbow.
    e) **TRUE**

44. a) **TRUE**
    b) **TRUE**
    c) **TRUE**
    d) **FALSE** In the femoral triangle the vein is medial to the artery. It crosses behind the artery to its lateral side as it enters the adductor canal.
    e) **TRUE** This is the midpoint between the anterior superior iliac spine and the pubic symphysis.

The Cardiovascular System

45. If the femoral artery is occluded in the middle of the thigh, blood can still pass into the lower extremity through the following arteries:
   a) internal pudendal
   b) iliolumbar
   c) profunda femoris
   d) lateral circumflex
   e) medial circumflex

46. The popliteal artery
   a) terminates at the upper border of the popliteus muscle
   b) has the tibial and common peroneal arteries as the terminal branches
   c) is covered superficially by the popliteal vein
   d) is crossed by the tibial nerve
   e) pulsation cannot be felt

47. The posterior tibial artery
   a) divides into the lateral and medial plantar arteries
   b) continues into the foot as the dorsalis pedis artery
   c) is accompanied by the tibial nerve
   d) is accompanied by the deep peroneal nerve
   e) pulsation can be felt behind the lateral malleolus

48. The great saphenous vein
   a) is accompanied by the sural nerve
   b) passes through the saphenous opening to join the femoral vein
   c) is connected to the deep veins by valveless channels
   d) lies in front of the medial malleolus
   e) may be distinguished from the femoral vein at operation by not having any tributary in its upper part

The Cardiovascular System

45. a) **FALSE**
    b) **FALSE**
    c) **TRUE**
    d) **TRUE**
    e) **TRUE**

46. a) **FALSE** It terminates at the lower border of popliteus.
    b) **FALSE** The terminal branches are the anterior and posterior tibial arteries.
    c) **TRUE**
    d) **TRUE**
    e) **FALSE** Pulsation of the artery can be felt on deep palpation.

47. a) **TRUE** Behind the medial malleolus.
    b) **FALSE** The dorsalis pedis is a continuation of the anterior tibial artery.
    c) **TRUE**
    d) **FALSE** This nerve accompanies the anterior tibial artery.
    e) **FALSE** Pulsation is felt behind the medial malleolus.

48. a) **FALSE** It is accompanied by the saphenous nerve.
    b) **TRUE**
    c) **FALSE** The connecting channels have valves.
    d) **TRUE** This is a constant position for the vein.
    e) **FALSE** The two veins may be distinguished by the saphenous having a number of tributaries. The only tributary for the femoral vein is the saphenous vein.

The Cardiovascular System

Picture questions

Identify the numbered structures in the following illustrations from the choices given

Question 1
1. ___
2. ___
3. ___
4. ___
5. ___
6. ___
7. ___
8. ___
9. ___
10. ___
11. ___

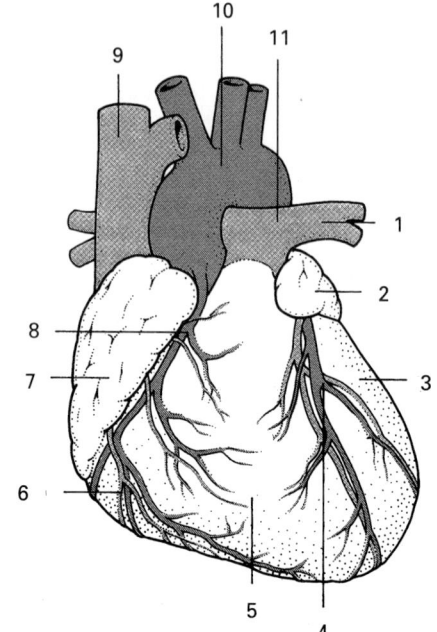

A. Right ventricle
B. Right coronary artery
C. Left pulmonary artery
D. Pulmonary trunk
E. Right atrium
F. Superior vena cava
G. Arch of aorta
H. Left ventricle
I. Small cardiac vein
J. Left auricle
K. Anterior descending (interventricular) branch of left coronary artery and great cardiac vein

286

The Cardiovascular System

Question 2
1. ____
2. ____
3. ____
4. ____
5. ____
6. ____

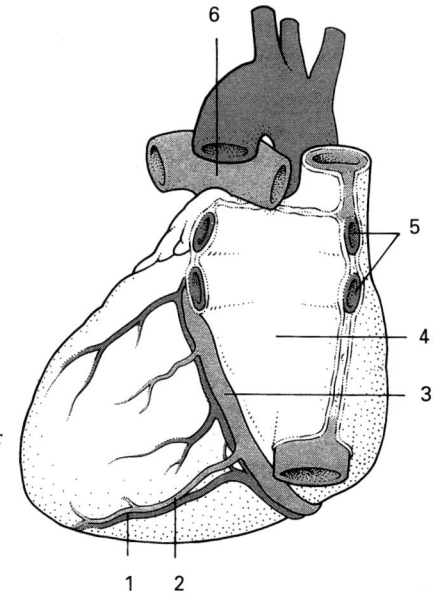

A. Coronary sinus
B. Left atrium
C. Middle cardiac vein
D. Right pulmonary veins
E. Posterior interventricular artery
F. Pulmonary trunk

Question 3
1. ____
2. ____
3. ____
4. ____
5. ____
6. ____
7. ____
8. ____
9. ____
10. ____
11. ____
12. ____

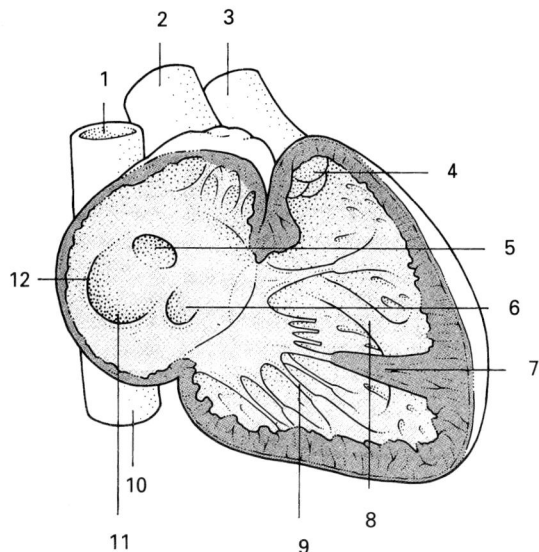

A. Superior vena cava
B. Opening of coronary sinus
C. Opening of inferior vena cava
D. Ascending aorta
E. Crista terminalis
F. Inferior vena cava
G. Pulmonary valve
H. Fossa ovalis
I. Pulmonary trunk
J. Papillary muscle
K. Moderator band
L. Chordae tendinae

Answers on page 301   287

The Cardiovascular System

Question 4
1. _____
2. _____
3. _____
4. _____
5. _____
6. _____
7. _____
8. _____

A. Inferior vena cava
B. Ascending aorta
C. Chordae tendinae
D. Right pulmonary veins
E. Mitral valve
F. Superior vena cava
G. Pulmonary trunk
H. Serous pericardium

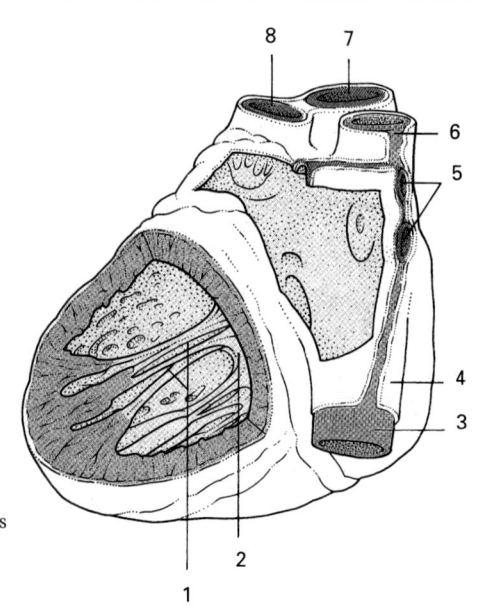

The Cardiovascular System

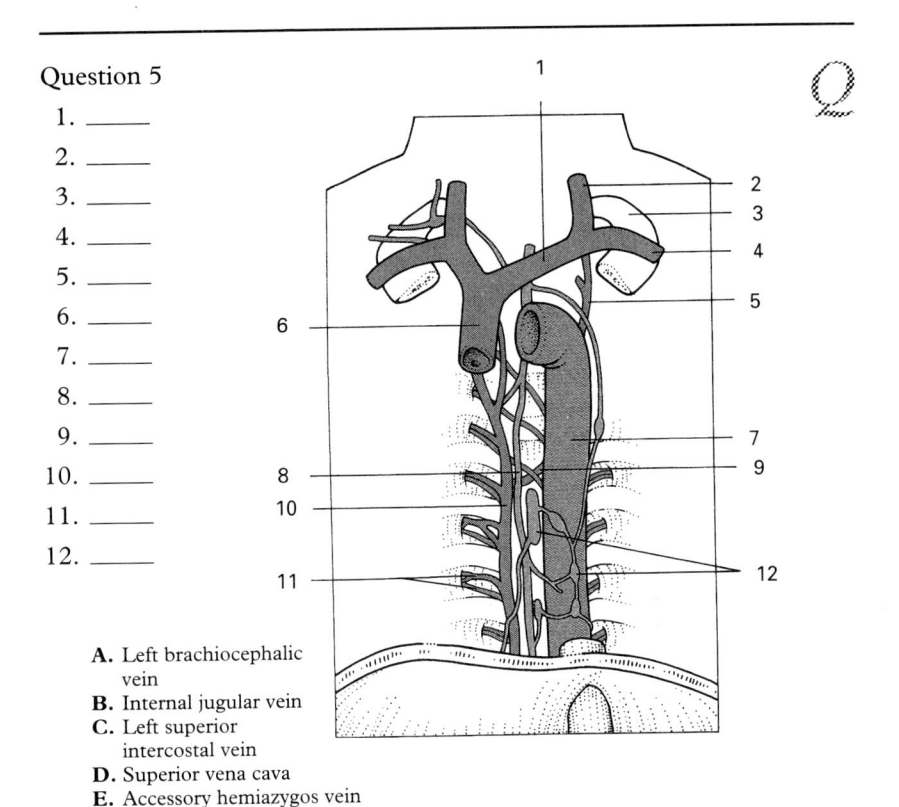

Question 5

1. ____
2. ____
3. ____
4. ____
5. ____
6. ____
7. ____
8. ____
9. ____
10. ____
11. ____
12. ____

A. Left brachiocephalic vein
B. Internal jugular vein
C. Left superior intercostal vein
D. Superior vena cava
E. Accessory hemiazygos vein
F. Azygos vein
G. Lymph nodes
H. 1st rib
I. Subclavian vein
J. Descending thoracic aorta
K. Thoracic duct
L. Posterior intercostal artery and vein

The Cardiovascular System

Question 6
1. ____
2. ____
3. ____
4. ____
5. ____
6. ____
7. ____
8. ____
9. ____
10. ____
11. ____
12. ____
13. ____
14. ____
15. ____

A. Ureter
B. Left renal vein
C. Inferior mesenteric artery
D. Inferior vena cava
E. Coeliac trunk
F. Abdominal aorta
G. Gonadal artery and vein
H. External iliac artery and vein
I. Left common iliac vein
J. Right common iliac artery
K. Inferior phrenic artery
L. Left crus
M. Internal iliac artery
N. Superior mesenteric artery
O. Diaphragm

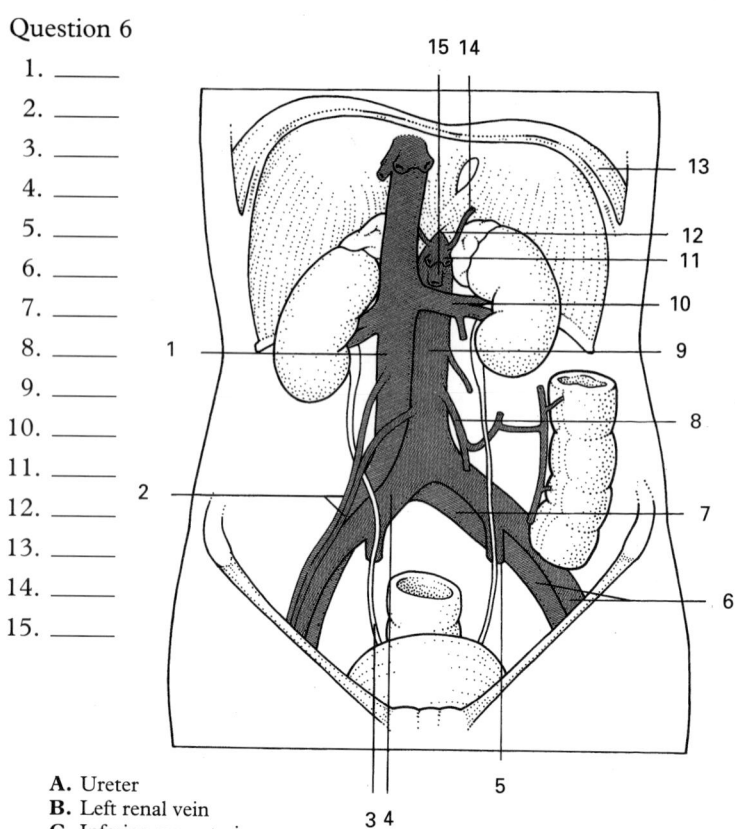

The Cardiovascular System

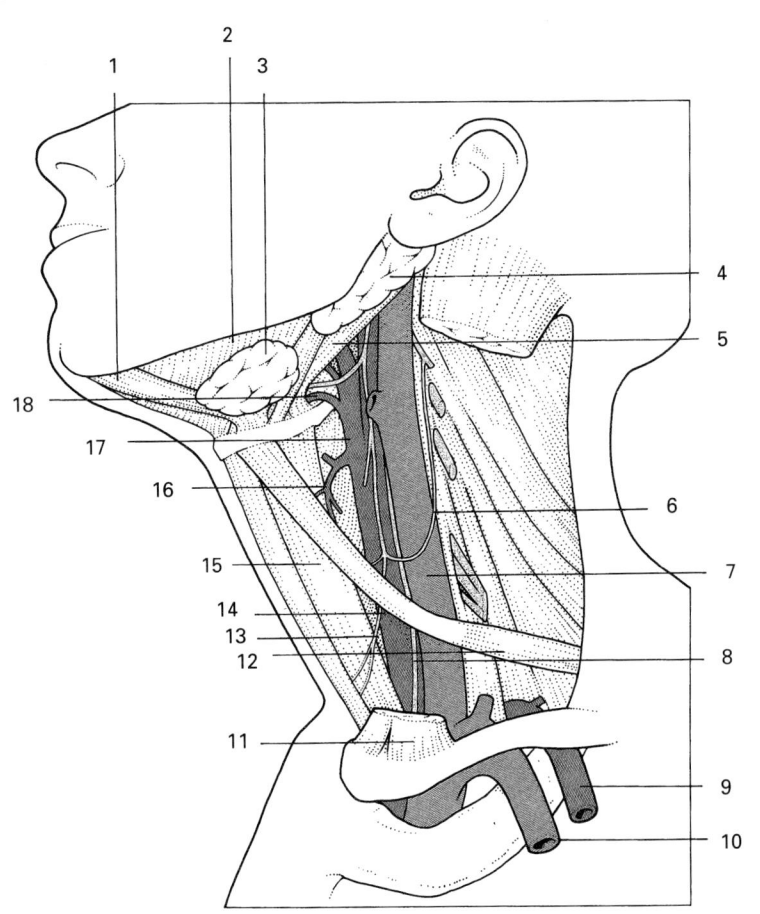

Question 7

1. ___	5. ___	9. ___	13. ___	17. ___
2. ___	6. ___	10. ___	14. ___	18. ___
3. ___	7. ___	11. ___	15. ___	
4. ___	8. ___	12. ___	16. ___	

A. Parotid gland
B. Ansa cervicalis
C. Vagus nerve
D. Anterior belly of digastric muscle
E. Mylohyoid muscle
F. Posterior belly of digastric muscle
G. Internal jugular vein
H. Submandibular gland
I. Subclavian artery
J. Omohyoid muscle
K. External carotid artery
L. Lingual artery
M. Subclavian vein
N. Sternothyroid muscle
O. Sternomastoid muscle (cut)
P. Superior thyroid artery
Q. Sternohyoid muscle
R. Common carotid artery

Answers on pages 302 and 303

The Cardiovascular System

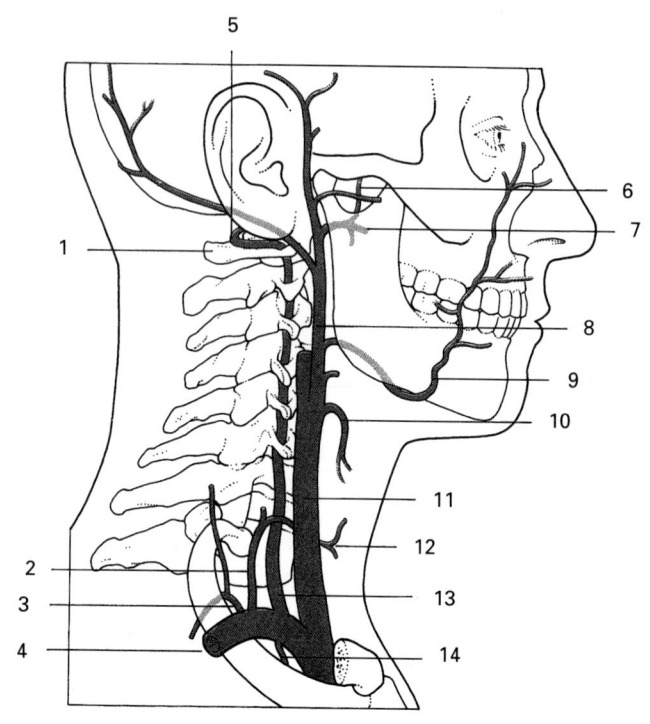

Question 8

1. ____
2. ____
3. ____
4. ____
5. ____
6. ____
7. ____
8. ____
9. ____
10. ____
11. ____
12. ____
13. ____
14. ____

A. Inferior thyroid artery
B. Atlas
C. Subclavian artery
D. Internal thoracic artery
E. Vertebral artery
F. Costocervical trunk
G. Maxillary artery
H. Vertebral artery
I. Facial artery
J. External carotid artery
K. Common carotid artery
L. Thyrocervical trunk
M. Middle meningeal artery
N. Superior thyroid artery

The Cardiovascular System

Question 9

1. ____
2. ____
3. ____

A. Middle cerebral artery
B. Anterior cerebral artery
C. Posterior cerebral artery

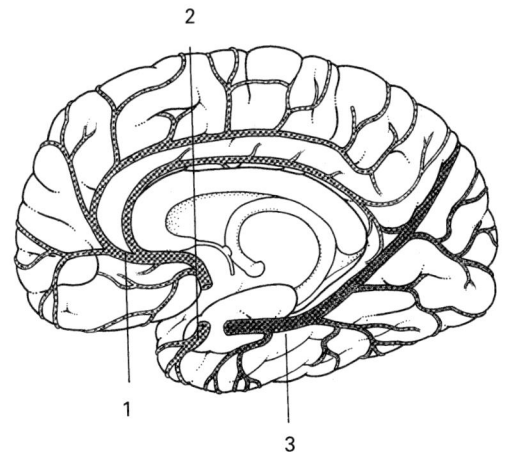

Question 10

1. ____
2. ____
3. ____

A. Branches from anterior cerebral artery
B. Middle cerebral artery
C. Branches from posterior cerebral artery

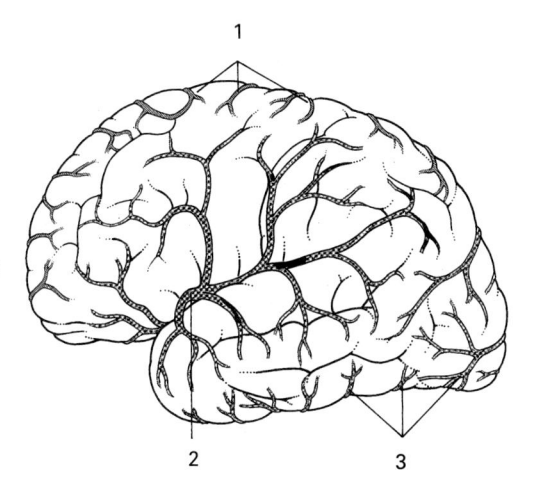

Answers on pages 303 and 304

The Cardiovascular System

Question 11

1. _____
2. _____
3. _____
4. _____
5. _____
6. _____
7. _____
8. _____
9. _____
10. _____
11. _____
12. _____
13. _____
14. _____

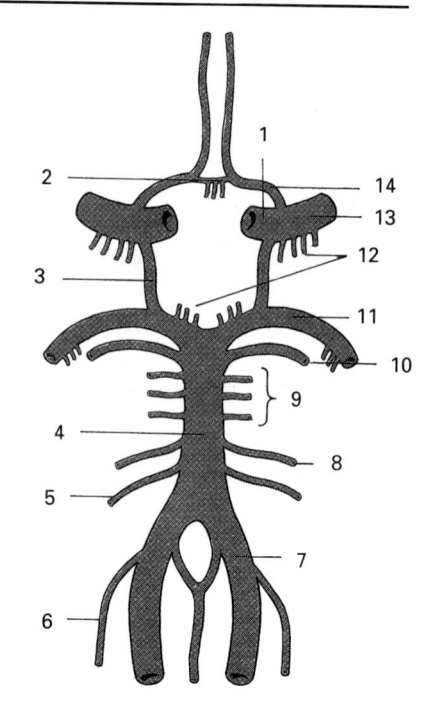

A. Internal carotid artery
B. Posterior inferior cerebellar artery
C. Superior cerebellar artery
D. Central arteries
E. Anterior cerebral artery
F. Anterior communicating artery
G. Anterior inferior cerebellar artery
H. Labyrinthine artery
I. Posterior communicating artery
J. Middle cerebral artery
K. Basilar artery
L. Vertebral artery
M. Posterior cerebral artery
N. Pontine branches

The Cardiovascular System

Question 12

1. _____
2. _____
3. _____
4. _____
5. _____
6. _____
7. _____

A. Jejunal and ileal arteries
B. Right colic artery
C. Left colic artery (from inferior mesenteric)
D. Middle colic artery
E. Marginal artery
F. Superior mesenteric artery
G. Ileocolic artery

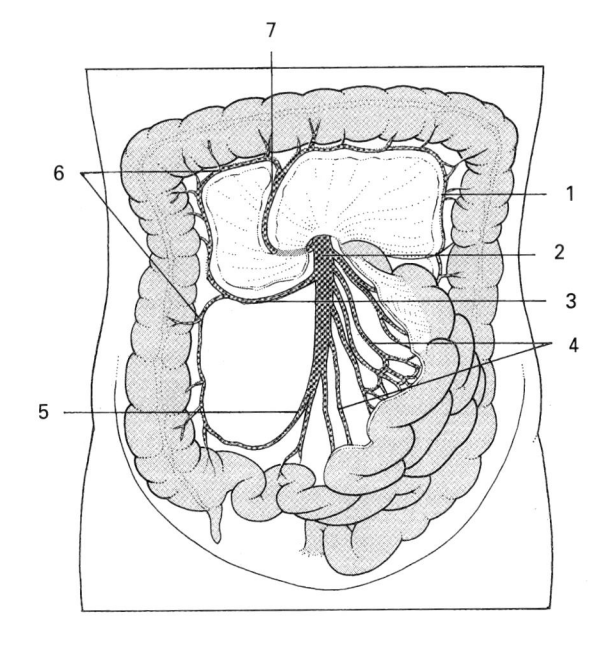

The Cardiovascular System

Question 13

1. ____
2. ____
3. ____
4. ____
5. ____
6. ____
7. ____
8. ____
9. ____
10. ____
11. ____
12. ____
13. ____
14. ____
15. ____

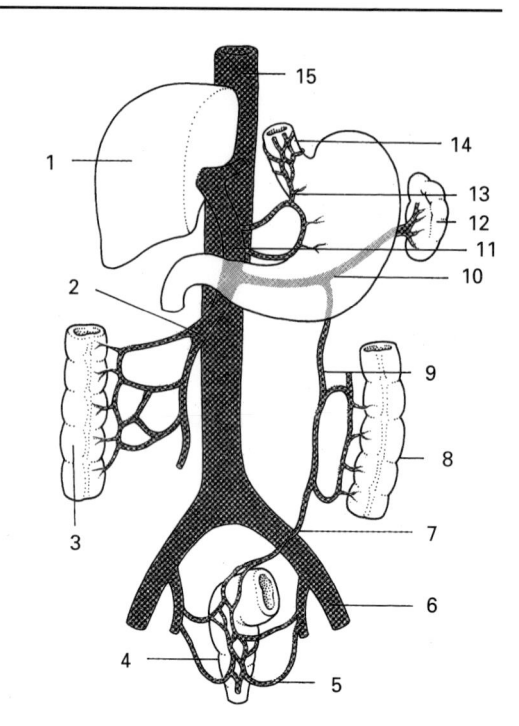

A. Inferior vena cava
B. Liver
C. Veins draining to azygos vein
D. Superior mesenteric vein
E. External iliac vein
F. Descending colon
G. Rectum and anal canal
H. Ascending colon
I. Left gastric vein
J. Inferior mesenteric vein
K. Spleen
L. Superior rectal vein
M. Portal vein
N. Inferior rectal vein
O. Splenic vein

The Cardiovascular System

Question 14
1. _____
2. _____
3. _____
4. _____
5. _____
6. _____
7. _____
8. _____

A. Internal iliac artery
B. Urinary bladder
C. Vaginal artery
D. Superior gluteal artery
E. Superior vesical artery
F. Uterine artery
G. Uterus
H. Ureter

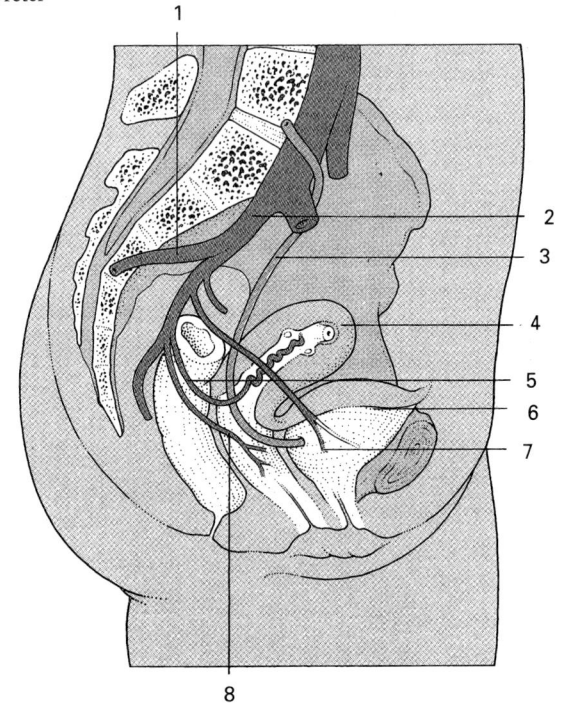

The Cardiovascular System

Question 15
1. ____
2. ____
3. ____
4. ____
5. ____
6. ____
7. ____
8. ____
9. ____
10. ____
11. ____
12. ____
13. ____

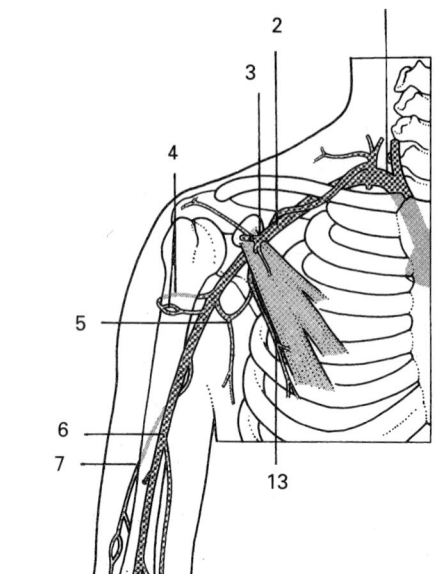

A. Subscapular artery
B. Profunda brachii artery
C. Superficial palmar arch
D. Ulnar artery
E. Lateral thoracic artery
F. Subclavian artery
G. Thoracoacromial artery
H. Brachial artery
I. Deep palmar arch
J. Axillary artery
K. Anterior and posterior circumflex humeral arteries
L. Common interosseus artery
M. Radial artery

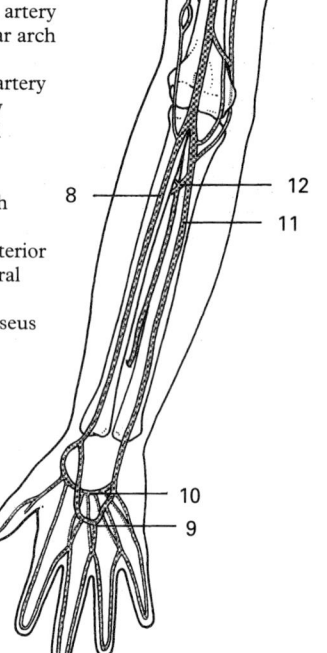

The Cardiovascular System

Question 16
1. ___
2. ___
3. ___
4. ___
5. ___
6. ___
7. ___
8. ___
9. ___
10. ___
11. ___

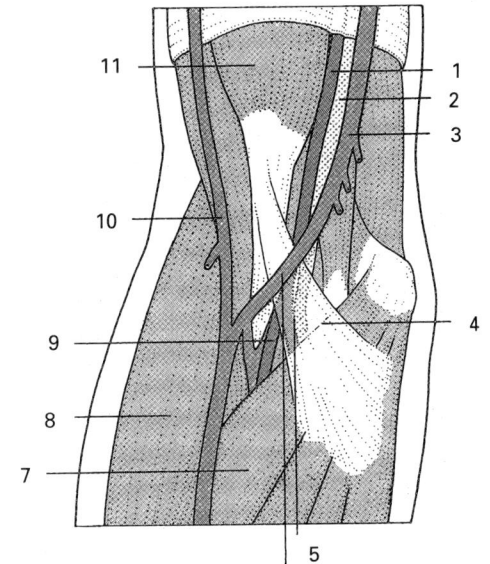

A. Radial artery
B. Brachioradialis muscle
C. Basilic vein
D. Median cubital vein
E. Brachial artery
F. Ulnar artery
G. Biceps muscle
H. Cephalic vein
I. Pronator teres
J. Median nerve
K. Bicipital aponeurosis

Answers on pages 305 and 306 299

The Cardiovascular System

Question 17
1. ____
2. ____
3. ____
4. ____
5. ____
6. ____

A. Superficial external pudendal vein
B. Great saphenous vein
C. Superficial external iliac vein
D. Femoral vein
E. Medial malleolus
F. Superficial epigastric vein

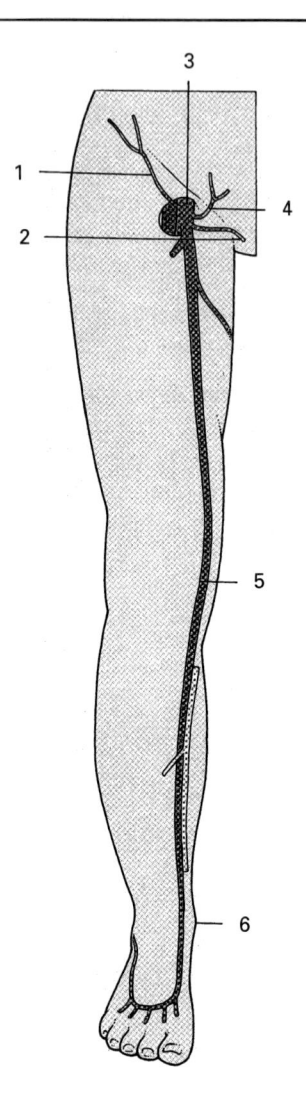

The Cardiovascular System

Picture questions A

Question 1
1. **C** Left pulmonary artery
2. **J** Left auricle
3. **H** Left ventricle
4. **K** Anterior descending (interventricular) branch of left coronary artery and great cardiac vein
5. **A** Right ventricle
6. **I** Small cardiac vein
7. **E** Right atrium
8. **B** Right coronary artery
9. **F** Superior vena cava
10. **G** Arch of aorta
11. **D** Pulmonary trunk

Question 2
1. **E** Posterior interventricular artery
2. **C** Middle cardiac vein
3. **A** Coronary sinus
4. **B** Left atrium
5. **D** Right pulmonary veins
6. **F** Pulmonary trunk

Question 3
1. **A** Superior vena cava
2. **D** Ascending aorta
3. **I** Pulmonary trunk
4. **G** Pulmonary valve
5. **H** Fossa ovalis
6. **B** Opening of coronary sinus
7. **J** Papillary muscle
8. **K** Moderator band
9. **L** Chordae tendinae
10. **F** Inferior vena cava
11. **C** Opening of inferior vena cava
12. **E** Crista terminalis

The Cardiovascular System

A Question 4
1. **C** Chordae tendinae
2. **E** Mitral valve
3. **A** Inferior vena cava
4. **H** Serous pericardium
5. **D** Right pulmonary veins
6. **F** Superior vena cava
7. **B** Ascending aorta
8. **G** Pulmonary trunk

Question 5
1. **A** Left brachiocephalic vein
2. **B** Internal jugular vein
3. **H** 1st rib
4. **I** Subclavian vein
5. **C** Left superior intercostal vein
6. **D** Superior vena cava
7. **J** Descending thoracic aorta
8. **K** Thoracic duct
9. **E** Accessory hemiazygos vein
10. **F** Azygos vein
11. **L** Posterior intercostal artery and vein
12. **G** Lymph nodes

Question 6
1. **D** Inferior vena cava
2. **G** Gonadal artery and vein
3. **A** Ureter
4. **J** Right common iliac artery
5. **M** Internal iliac artery
6. **H** External iliac artery and vein
7. **I** Left common iliac vein
8. **C** Inferior mesenteric artery
9. **F** Abdominal aorta
10. **B** Left renal vein
11. **E** Coeliac trunk
12. **L** Left crus
13. **O** Diaphragm
14. **K** Inferior phrenic artery
15. **N** Superior mesenteric artery

The Cardiovascular System

Question 7
1. **D** Anterior belly of digastric muscle
2. **E** Mylohyoid muscle
3. **H** Submandibular gland
4. **A** Parotid gland
5. **F** Posterior belly of digastric muscle
6. **B** Ansa cervicalis
7. **G** Internal jugular vein
8. **C** Vagus nerve
9. **I** Subclavian artery
10. **M** Subclavian vein
11. **O** Sternomastoid muscle (cut)
12. **J** Omohyoid muscle
13. **N** Sternothyroid muscle
14. **R** Common carotid artery
15. **Q** Sternohyoid muscle
16. **P** Superior thyroid artery
17. **K** External carotid artery
18. **L** Lingual artery

Question 8
1. **B** Atlas
2. **L** Thyrocervical trunk
3. **F** Costocervical trunk
4. **C** Subclavian artery
5. **E** Vertebral artery
6. **M** Middle meningeal artery
7. **G** Maxillary artery
8. **J** External carotid artery
9. **I** Facial artery
10. **N** Superior thyroid artery
11. **K** Common carotid artery
12. **A** Inferior thyroid artery
13. **H** Vertebral artery
14. **D** Internal thoracic artery

Question 9
1. **B** Anterior cerebral artery
2. **A** Middle cerebral artery
3. **C** Posterior cerebral artery

The Cardiovascular System

Question 10
1. **A** Branches from the anterior cerebral artery
2. **B** Middle cerebral artery
3. **C** Branches from the posterior cerebral artery

Question 11
1. **A** Internal carotid artery
2. **F** Anterior communicating artery
3. **I** Posterior communicating artery
4. **K** Basilar artery
5. **G** Anterior inferior cerebellar artery
6. **B** Posterior inferior cerebellar artery
7. **L** Vertebral artery
8. **H** Labyrinthine artery
9. **N** Pontine branches
10. **C** Superior cerebellar artery
11. **M** Posterior cerebral artery
12. **D** Central arteries
13. **J** Middle cerebral artery
14. **E** Anterior cerebral artery

Question 12
1. **C** Left colic artery (from inferior mesenteric)
2. **F** Superior mesenteric artery
3. **B** Right colic artery
4. **A** Jejunal and ileal arteries
5. **G** Ileocolic artery
6. **E** Marginal artery
7. **D** Middle colic artery

The Cardiovascular System

Question 13
1. **B** Liver
2. **D** Superior mesenteric vein
3. **H** Ascending colon
4. **G** Rectum and anal canal
5. **N** Inferior rectal vein
6. **E** External iliac vein
7. **L** Superior rectal vein
8. **F** Descending colon
9. **J** Inferior mesenteric vein
10. **O** Splenic vein
11. **M** Portal vein
12. **K** Spleen
13. **I** Left gastric vein
14. **C** Veins draining to azygos vein
15. **A** Inferior vena cava

Question 14
1. **D** Superior gluteal artery
2. **A** Internal iliac artery
3. **H** Ureter
4. **G** Uterus
5. **F** Uterine artery
6. **B** Urinary bladder
7. **E** Superior vesical artery
8. **C** Vaginal artery

Question 15
1. **F** Subclavian artery
2. **J** Axillary artery
3. **G** Thoracoacromial artery
4. **K** Anterior and posterior circumflex humeral arteries
5. **A** Subscapular artery
6. **H** Brachial artery
7. **B** Profunda brachii artery
8. **M** Radial artery
9. **C** Superficial palmar arch
10. **I** Deep palmar arch
11. **D** Ulnar artery
12. **L** Common interosseus artery
13. **E** Lateral thoracic artery

The Cardiovascular System

A Question 16
1. **E** Brachial artery
2. **J** Median nerve
3. **C** Basilic vein
4. **K** Bicipital aponeurosis
5. **F** Ulnar artery
6. **D** Median cubital vein
7. **I** Pronator teres
8. **B** Brachioradialis muscle
9. **A** Radial artery
10. **H** Cephalic vein
11. **G** Biceps muscle

Question 17
1. **C** Superficial external iliac vein
2. **A** Superficial external pudendal vein
3. **D** Femoral vein
4. **F** Superficial epigastric vein
5. **B** Great saphenous vein
6. **E** Medial malleolus

The Cardiovascular System

Clinical problems

1. A 55-year-old man was admitted to hospital with excruciating chest pain, nausea and vomiting and severe shortness of breath. His pulse was weak and rapid, blood pressure low, and respiration noisy and gasping. He used to suffer from chest pain that radiated into the left arm. Myocardial infarction (heart attack) was confirmed by ECG. In spite of treatment by specialists in the coronary care unit the patient died two hours after admission. Autopsy revealed marked narrowing of both the coronary arteries and most of their branches due to atherosclerosis. What is the arterial supply of the heart and where do these arteries originate from? To what extent is the statement that the right coronary artery supplies the right heart and the left coronary artery the left heart true? What is the blood supply of the interatrial and interventricular septa? What is the blood supply of the conducting system? Are coronary arteries end-arteries?

The Cardiovascular System

A Clinical problems

1. The right and left coronary arteries are medium-sized arteries and arise from the right and left aortic sinuses of the ascending aorta just distal to the aortic valve. Typically, the right coronary artery supplies the right atrium and the right ventricle, with the exception of the left part of the sternocostal surface of the right ventricle, which is supplied by the anterior descending (anterior interventricular) branch of the left coronary artery. The left coronary artery supplies the left atrium and the left ventricle, with the exception of the right part of the diaphragmatic surface of the left ventricle, which is supplied by the inferior descending (posterior interventricular) branch of the right coronary artery. The interatrial septum is usually supplied by the right coronary artery, whereas the interventricular septum is supplied by both the coronaries through their interventricular branches, with the left carrying the major share. The blood supply of the conducting system is variable. The sinoatrial node is supplied by the right coronary artery in about 60% of individuals, with the circumflex branch of the left coronary supplying the rest. However, the arterioventricular node and the proximal part of the arterioventricular bundle receive their blood supply in about 90% of cases from the right coronary artery. Structurally, the coronary arteries are not end-arteries; their branches do anastomose (communicate). However, collateral circulation in these anastomoses is absent or inadequate, and blockage of a branch of one artery will produce necrosis of the area it supplies. The area of necrosis is known as an infarct.

The Cardiovascular System

2. Valvular diseases of the heart can be produced as a complication of rheumatic fever, which is still common in many regions of Asia and Africa. Mitral stenosis is a condition where there is obstruction to the flow of blood from the left atrium to the left ventricle. In which phase of the cardiac cycle does blood flow from the atrium to the ventricle? Where is the mitral sound best heard? Mitral stenosis will increase the left atrial pressure and produce left atrial hypertrophy. Which structure is closely related to the posterior aspect of the left atrium? Pooling of blood in the pulmonary circulation in mitral stenosis will produce pulmonary hypertension and right ventricular hypertrophy. What is the normal surface anatomy of the right ventricle? Right ventricular hypertrophy is often characterised by a less prominent (tapping) apex beat. Which chamber of the heart contributes to the apex beat? Where is it usually located? In which condition may the apex beat be shifted downwards and outwards, where it will also be more prominent than normal?

3. A child who presented with symptoms of breathlessness on exertion and retarded growth was found to have a continuous machinery murmur best heard in the pulmonary area. Diagnosis of patent ductus arteriosus was made. What is the ductus arteriosus? What is its function? Where does it develop from? Which nerve is closely related to the ductus? What happens to the ductus arteriosus after birth? In the fetus, which way does the blood flow in the ductus? If it remains patent after birth will the flow maintain the same direction? Name two other areas where there are similar connections in the fetal circulation. What happens to them after birth?

Answers on page 310

The Cardiovascular System

2. Blood flows from the left atrium to the left ventricle in ventricular diastole. A presystolic murmur is a characteristic feature of mitral stenosis and it will be best heard at the apex of the heart. The oesophagus lies closely behind the left atrium, separated only by the oblique sinus of the pericardium. Normally there is an indentation on the oesophagus produced by the left atrium and this is accentuated in left atrial hypertrophy. The border of the right ventricle extends from the third to the sixth costal cartilage along the lateral border of the sternum. This border may be shifted outwards in right ventricular hypertrophy. The right ventricle is the anterior chamber and hence when it enlarges the left ventricle lies further away from the anterior chest wall. This will result in a less prominent apex beat. The apex of the heart is formed entirely by the left ventricle. Normally the apex beat is located in the fifth intercostal space inside the midclavicular line on the left side. Left ventricular hypertrophy, as might happen in aortic valve stenosis, shifts the apex beat downwards and to the left and also makes it very prominent.

3. The ductus arteriosus connects the left pulmonary artery to the arch of the aorta just distal to the origin of the left subclavian artery. In the fetus, it functions to shunt blood from the pulmonary trunk to the aorta, bypassing the lungs. It is developed from the left sixth aortic arch connecting the ventral and dorsal aorta. The left recurrent laryngeal nerve winds round it. After birth the ductus goes into spasm and eventually obliterates to give rise to the ligamentum arteriosum. In the fetus, blood flows from the pulmonary trunk to the aorta as the right-sided pressure is higher. After birth there is reversal of pressure, and if the ductus remains patent blood flow will be from the aorta to the pulmonary artery.

There are two other connections in the fetal circulation which obliterate soon after birth. The ductus venosus becomes the ligamentum venosum. In the fetus, the ductus venosus connects the umbilical vein to the inferior vena cava, bypassing the liver. The foramen ovale on the interatrial septum shunts blood from the right atrium to the left atrium in the fetus. It becomes the fossa ovalis after birth.

The Cardiovascular System

4. Varicose veins are dilated tortuous veins usually seen in the lower limb. What is the mechanism of venous return in the lower limb? How are varicose veins produced?

The Cardiovascular System

4. The veins of the lower extremity are in two sets, superficial and deep. The long and short saphenous veins are the two main superficial veins. The long saphenous vein is formed from the medial aspect of the dorsal venous arch of the foot. It lies in front of the medial malleolus and behind the medial condyle of the femur as it ascends towards its termination at the sapheno-femoral junction. The vein passes through the saphenous opening, which is 3–4 cm below and lateral to the pubic tubercle, in the deep fascia, before joining the femoral vein. It has a number of tributaries throughout its course including its terminal portion. The short saphenous vein usually terminates in the popliteal vein. The deep veins, lying deep to the deep fascia, accompany the main arteries of the leg. The superficial veins are connected to the deep veins by perforating veins as well as at their termination at the sapheno-femoral junction. Normally blood flows from the superficial veins to the deep veins. From the deep veins blood is pumped upwards against gravity by the calf muscles. Muscle weakness and deep fascia stretching will affect this pump. Back flow from deep to superficial veins is prevented by valves. There are valves at the sapheno-femoral and sapheno-popliteal junctions and in many other locations. Valves can withstand pressure of up to 90 mm Hg exerted by the column of blood on standing. When the valves become incompetent, blood will flow back from the deep veins to the superficial making them varicose. Varicosity is also predisposed to by obstruction to the venous blood flow produced by tumours and pregnancy as well as by deep vein thrombosis.

The Urinary System

The Urinary System

THE URINARY SYSTEM

True/False

1. **Regarding the right kidney:**
   a) it lies behind the liver
   b) it is related to the pleural cavity, separated by the diaphragm
   c) the hilum is just above the transpyloric plane
   d) the ureter lies anteriorly at the hilum
   e) more than one renal artery enters the hilum

2. **The following statements about the kidneys are true:**
   a) the cortex contains the glomeruli
   b) the cortex contains the loops of Henle
   c) a major calyx surrounds the apex of a pyramid
   d) they move with respiration
   e) there is perirenal fat outside the renal capsule

3. **The left renal vein**
   a) crosses the aorta anteriorly just above the origin of the superior mesenteric artery
   b) lies posterior to the left renal artery
   c) lies posterior to the body of the pancreas
   d) has the left gonadal vein opening into it
   e) is shorter than the right vein

4. **The ureters**
   a) are about 25 cm long
   b) lie 2 cm lateral to the tips of the lumbar transverse processes
   c) cross the bifurcation of the aorta
   d) are supplied mainly by the lumbar arteries
   e) are constricted halfway along their course

The Urinary System

THE URINARY SYSTEM

1. a) **TRUE**   The two are separated by the hepatorenal pouch.
   b) **TRUE**   Both kidneys are related to the pleural cavities.
   c) **FALSE**   The hilum of the right kidney lies just below the transpyloric plane.
   d) **FALSE**   The ureter lies posteriorly at the hilum.
   e) **TRUE**   There are usually three branches of the renal artery entering the hilum of the kidney.

2. a) **TRUE**   The cortex also contains the proximal and distal convoluted tubules.
   b) **FALSE**   The loops of Henle are found in the medulla.
   c) **FALSE**   Minor calyces surround the pyramid apices.
   d) **TRUE**   They move down during inspiration and up during expiration.
   e) **TRUE**   Perirenal fat lies between the renal fascia and the capsule of the kidney.

3. a) **FALSE**   It crosses the aorta anteriorly but below the origin of the superior mesenteric artery.
   b) **FALSE**   The renal vein lies anteriorly.
   c) **TRUE**   The pancreas crosses in front of the kidney.
   d) **TRUE**   The right gonadal vein opens directly into the inferior vena cava.
   e) **FALSE**   The left vein is longer.

4. a) **TRUE**   Same length as the oesophagus.
   b) **FALSE**   The ureters lie on the lumbar transverse processes. The structures are separated by the psoas major muscles.
   c) **FALSE**   They cross in front of the bifurcation of the common iliac arteries.
   d) **FALSE**   The ureters are supplied by all the arteries along their course, i.e. the renal, gonadal, internal iliac and inferior vesical arteries.
   e) **FALSE**   The ureter is constricted at its commencement at the pelvi-ureteric junction, where it crosses the common iliac artery and just before it enters the bladder.

The Urinary System

5. **The ureter**
   a) develops from the mesonephric duct
   b) passes below the uterine artery
   c) crosses above the ductus deferens
   d) has columnar epithelium
   e) adheres to the overlying peritoneum

6. **Regarding the urinary bladder:**
   a) it is derived entirely from endoderm
   b) its base is completely covered by peritoneum
   c) its motor supply is from both sympathetic and parasympathetic systems
   d) its only sensory supply is from the sympathetic system
   e) it is lined by transitional epithelium

7. **The following statements about the urinary bladder are true:**
   a) when empty the trigonal mucosa has folds
   b) the interureteric ridge forms the upper border (base) of the trigone
   c) a smooth muscle sphincter is present at the bladder neck in the male
   d) the ductus deferens lies medial to the seminal vesicle on the posterior surface
   e) it lies in the abdomen in the infant

8. **Concerning the male urethra:**
   a) the prostatic urethra receives the ejaculatory duct
   b) the colliculus seminalis is in the membranous part
   c) the membranous part is the least dilatable
   d) the membranous part is surrounded by the sphincter urethrae (external sphincter)
   e) the bulbar part lies in the corpus cavernosum

The Urinary System

5. a) **TRUE** The collecting ducts of the kidney also develop from the mesonephric duct.
   b) **TRUE** The ureter then runs forward, lateral to the lateral fornix of the vagina, to enter the bladder.
   c) **FALSE** The ductus deferens crosses the ureter superiorly.
   d) **FALSE** The epithelium is transitional.
   e) **TRUE** This fact is useful in exposing the ureter. As the parietal peritoneum is exposed, the ureter is seen stuck to its posterior surface.

6. a) **FALSE** The trigone is of mesodermal origin.
   b) **FALSE** Peritoneum covers only the upper part of the base in both male and female.
   c) **FALSE** Only parasympathetic fibres (pelvic splanchnic nerves) have motor functions.
   d) **FALSE** There are also sensory parasympathetic fibres.
   e) **TRUE** This allows the bladder to distend.

7. a) **FALSE** This is the only part without folds.
   b) **TRUE** The ureters open at either end of this ridge. The apex of the trigone is where the bladder opens into the urethra.
   c) **TRUE** It is called the sphincter vesicae or internal sphincter and it prevents seminal fluid from entering the bladder during ejaculation.
   d) **TRUE** The common ejaculatory duct is formed from the ductus deferens and the duct of the seminal vesicle.
   e) **TRUE** The bladder becomes pelvic at about the age of six.

8. a) **TRUE** The ducts of the prostate gland also open into this part of the urethra.
   b) **FALSE** The colliculus seminalis, part of the urethral crest, is in the prostatic urethra.
   c) **TRUE** This part is about 1.5 cm in length. The male urethra is narrowest at the bladder neck, in the membraneous part, at the proximal end of the navicular fossa and at the external meatus.
   d) **TRUE** It is made of striated muscle and is concerned with control of micturition.
   e) **FALSE** It is in the corpus spongiosum of the penis.

The Urinary System

9. **The female urethra**
   a) lies on the anterior wall of the vagina
   b) opens into the vestibule
   c) is about 4 cm long
   d) does not possess an external sphincter as in the male
   e) is lined by transitional epithelium throughout

10. **Regarding urinary continence:**
    a) the intrinsic external sphincter (striated muscle) plays an important role
    b) the external sphincter is innervated by the S2–S4 spinal cord segments
    c) the internal sphincter (smooth muscle sphincter at the bladder neck) prevents semen entering the bladder during ejaculation
    d) transurethral prostatic resection results in incontinence
    e) it is affected by spinal cord injuries

The Urinary System

9. a) **TRUE** It is embedded in the vaginal wall.
   b) **TRUE** The vestibule lies between the labia minora.
   c) **TRUE**
   d) **FALSE** It has an external sphincter; however, it does not possess an internal sphincter at the bladder neck.
   e) **FALSE** The epithelium changes from transitional at the bladder neck, to pseudostratified columnar, to stratified squamous non-keratinised near the urethral meatus.

10. a) **TRUE**
    b) **TRUE** Through the pudendal nerve.
    c) **TRUE**
    d) **FALSE** Prostatectomy may damage the internal sphincter. However, urinary incontinence will not occur as long as the external sphincter remains intact.
    e) **TRUE** Normal filling and emptying is controlled by the sacral segments of the cord which in turn are controlled by higher centres.

The Urinary System

Picture questions

Identify the numbered structures in the following illustrations from the choices given

Question 1

1. ____
2. ____
3. ____
4. ____
5. ____
6. ____
7. ____
8. ____
9. ____
10. ____

A. Renal vein
B. Pelvis of ureter
C. Minor calyx
D. Cortex
E. Medulla
F. Renal artery
G. Ureter
H. Major calyx
I. Papilla
J. Pyramid

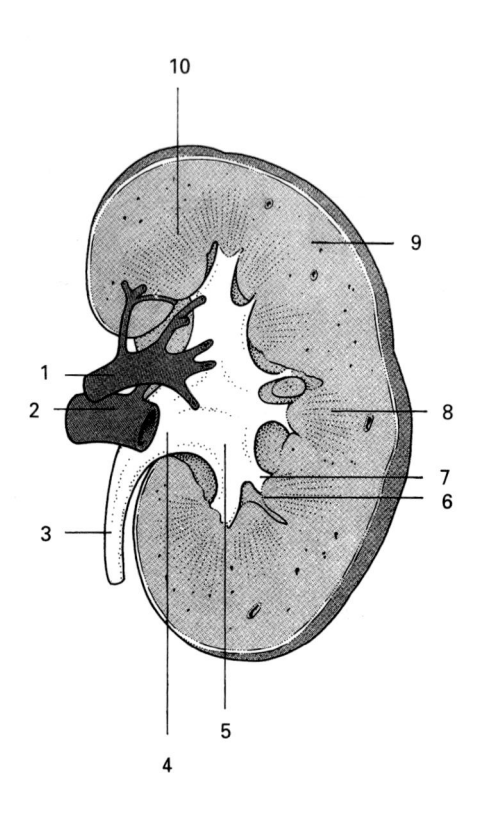

320

The Urinary System

Question 2
1. ___
2. ___
3. ___
4. ___
5. ___
6. ___
7. ___
8. ___
9. ___
10. ___

A. Ureter
B. Common iliac artery
C. Left gonadal vein
D. External iliac artery
E. Left renal vein
F. Right gonadal artery
G. Left psoas major
H. Inferior vena cava
I. Right gonadal vein
J. Bladder

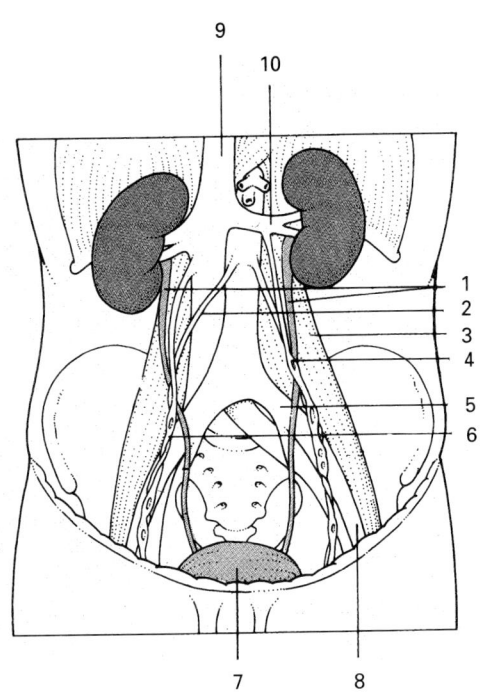

Answers on page 325 321

The Urinary System

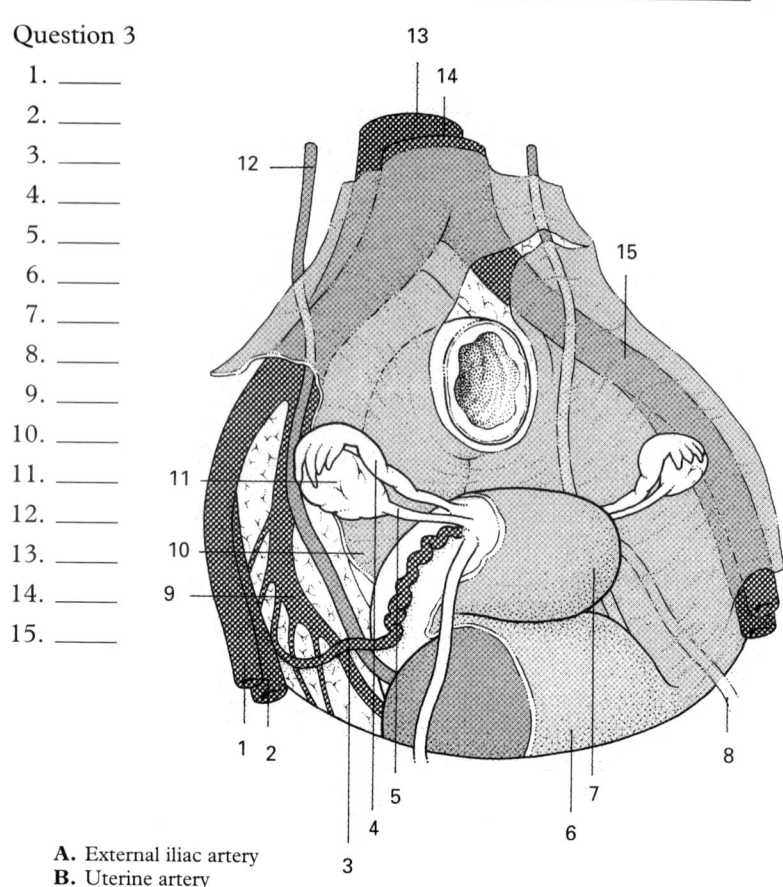

Question 3
1. ___
2. ___
3. ___
4. ___
5. ___
6. ___
7. ___
8. ___
9. ___
10. ___
11. ___
12. ___
13. ___
14. ___
15. ___

A. External iliac artery
B. Uterine artery
C. Ligament of ovary
D. Fundus of uterus
E. Common iliac artery
F. Superior vena cava
G. Ovary
H. Internal iliac artery
I. External iliac vein
J. Aorta
K. Uterine tube
L. Ureter
M. Bladder
N. Round ligament of uterus
O. Rectum

The Urinary System

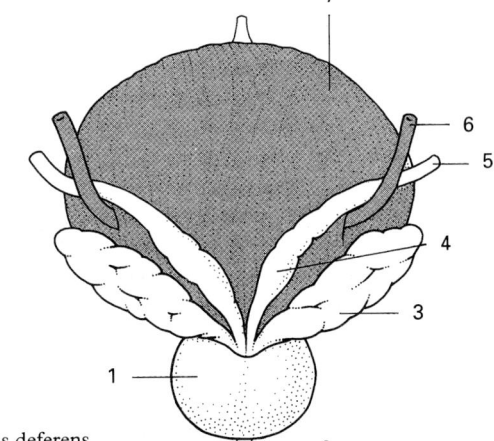

Question 4
1. ___
2. ___
3. ___
4. ___
5. ___
6. ___
7. ___

A. Bladder
B. Prostate
C. Seminal vesicle
D. Vas deferens
E. Ampulla of the vas deferens
F. Ureter
G. Urethra

The Urinary System

Question 5
1. ____
2. ____
3. ____
4. ____
5. ____
6. ____
7. ____
8. ____
9. ____
10. ____
11. ____
12. ____

A. Rectouterine pouch
B. Rectum
C. Retropubic space
D. Uterus
E. Urethra
F. Uterovesical pouch
G. Symphysis pubis
H. Vagina
I. Vestibule
J. Ureter
K. Cervix
L. Bladder

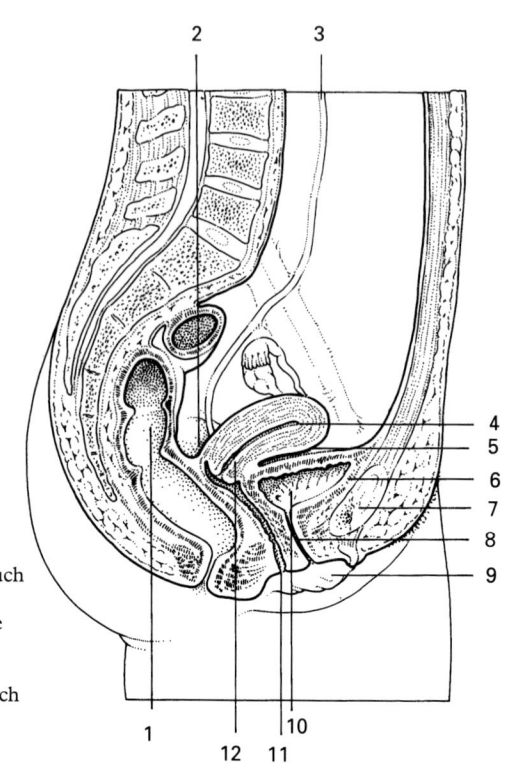

The Urinary System

Picture questions

Question 1
1. **F** Renal artery
2. **A** Renal vein
3. **G** Ureter
4. **B** Pelvis of ureter
5. **H** Major calyx
6. **I** Papilla
7. **C** Minor calyx
8. **J** Pyramid
9. **D** Cortex
10. **E** Medulla

Question 2
1. **A** Ureter
2. **F** Right gonadal artery
3. **G** Left psoas major
4. **C** Left gonadal vein
5. **B** Common iliac artery
6. **I** Right gonadal vein
7. **J** Bladder
8. **D** External iliac artery
9. **H** Inferior vena cava
10. **E** Left renal vein

Question 3
1. **A** External iliac artery
2. **I** External iliac vein
3. **B** Uterine artery
4. **K** Uterine tube
5. **C** Ligament of ovary
6. **M** Bladder
7. **D** Fundus of uterus
8. **N** Round ligament of uterus
9. **H** Internal iliac artery
10. **O** Rectum
11. **G** Ovary
12. **L** Ureter
13. **F** Superior vena cava
14. **J** Aorta
15. **E** Common iliac artery

325

The Urinary System

A Question 4
1. **B** Prostate
2. **G** Urethra
3. **C** Seminal vesicle
4. **E** Ampulla of the vas deferens
5. **D** Vas deferens
6. **F** Ureter
7. **A** Bladder

Question 5
1. **B** Rectum
2. **A** Rectouterine pouch
3. **J** Ureter
4. **D** Uterus
5. **F** Uterovesical pouch
6. **C** Retropubic space
7. **G** Symphysis pubis
8. **E** Urethra
9. **I** Vestibule
10. **L** Bladder
11. **H** Vagina
12. **K** Cervix

The Urinary System

Clinical problems

1. A 60-year-old male was admitted to hospital complaining of haematuria (blood in urine) and a dull ache in the left loin. On examination the left kidney was palpable and examination of the scrotum revealed a left sided varicocele which felt like a bag of worms. Further investigation revealed a malignant tumour in the kidney which had not spread to the lungs and bones. Is the normal kidney palpable? How does one distinguish a palpable spleen from a palpable left kidney? What is a varicocele? Is the varicocele in this case caused by the tumour in the kidney? By what route can tumour cells spread to the lung from the kidney? By what route may they reach the bones and liver? In this patient the affected kidney was removed through a lumbar incision below the twelfth rib. What structures will the surgeon come across on his way to the exposure of the kidney through this route? The surgeon will have to ligate and cut the structures at the hilum of the kidney during this procedure. What structures lie at the hilum and in what order?

The Urinary System

A Clinical problems

1. The normal kidney is not palpable. In this case it is enlarged due to the presence of the tumour. The kidney is bimanually palpable whereas an enlarged spleen is not. Moreover, the presence of palpable notches along the anterior border is a characteristic feature of an enlarged spleen. The renal tumour spreads into the renal vein and blocks the left testicular vein which drains into it. The testicular vein is formed from the pampiniform plexus of veins in the spermatic cord. When dilated and tortuous those form a varicocele. The tumour from the kidney can spread to the lung through the blood stream, through the inferior vena cava to the heart and then into the pulmonary trunk. It may also spread to bone and liver through blood.

   A lumbar incision is usually used to expose the kidney. The incision extends below the twelfth rib from the lateral border of the erector spinae to the anterior superior iliac spine. Latissimus dorsi and external oblique are incised, and deep to them internal oblique and transversus merging with the lumbar fascia. Subcostal nerves and vessels are encountered and the nerves are preserved. The surgeon makes every effort to avoid entering the pleural cavity, which extends up to the twelfth rib at this level. At the hilum of the kidney the renal vessels, the vein in front and the artery behind, will be ligated; the renal pelvis and the commencement of the ureter will be most posterior at the hilum.

The Urinary System

2. A ureteric calculus (stone) is a common cause of ureteric colic. The stone is always formed in the kidney. As it descends the ureter it causes colicky pain. There are five sites of anatomical narrowing where the stone may be arrested. What are these sites? When the stone is arrested at the pelviureteric junction the pain starts in the region of the kidney and radiates to the groin (loin to the groin). Which nerve transmits this pain? When the stone is arrested in the lower part of the ureter the pain is felt along the distribution of the genitofemoral nerve. What is the direction of this type of pain? In such cases, the testis becomes retracted. Why? When can a stone in the ureter be felt on physical examination?

3. Cystoscopy is a common urological examination. In this procedure, the cystoscope is passed into the bladder through the urethra and the interior of the bladder is examined. What structures/features may be distinguished inside the bladder? Instrumentation is more difficult in the male. What are the parts of the male urethra? What are the narrowest and least distensible parts of the male urethra?

The Urinary System

2. The ureter is constricted at the pelviureteric junction, at the pelvic brim where it crosses the termination of the common iliac artery, where it crosses the broad ligament in the female and the ductus deferens in the male, and finally at the ureteric orifice in the bladder. Ureteric pain is transmitted by the afferents accompanying the sympathetics and manifests as a referred pain along the region innervated by the upper lumbar nerves. Pain from the upper part of the ureter radiates along the L1 nerve distribution from loin to groin, whereas that from the lower part is transmitted by the genitofemoral nerve and radiates from the lower abdomen to the thigh (femoral branch) and to the scrotum or labium majus (genital branch). The testis in this type of colic is retracted by the spasm of the cremasteric muscle which is supplied by the genital branch of the genitofemoral nerve. In the female, the ureter lies close to the lateral fornix of the vagina (crossing below the uterine artery) and a ureteric stone at this site can be felt by vaginal examination.

3. The interior of the bladder and the three orifices, i.e. the two ureters and the urethra, are seen at cystoscopy. When the bladder is empty the ureteric orifices are 2.5 cm apart, but when distended for cystoscopic examination the distance may be about 5 cm. Between the ureters, the interureteric bar (ridge), a transverse fold of mucosa produced by underlying muscle, will be seen. The bladder mucosa is loosely adherent to the muscle and may be folded, except at the trigone where it is tightly adherent to the muscle and hence smooth in appearance. The trigone is bounded by the two ureteric orifices above and the urethra below.

The male urethra is 20 cm long and is divided into a prostatic (3 cm), membranous (2 cm), and spongy or penile urethra. It is narrowest at the bladder neck, in the membranous part and at the external meatus. The membranous urethra is the least distensible part of the male urethra.

The Reproductive System

The Reproductive System

THE REPRODUCTIVE SYSTEM

True/False

1. **Concerning the parts of the uterus:**
   a) the fundus is above the level of entry of the fallopian (uterine) tubes ____
   b) the body lies between the fundus and the cervix ____
   c) the cervix can be felt during rectal examination ____
   d) the entire cervix is intravaginal ____
   e) the external os communicates with the body and the cervix ____

2. **Among the structures that hold the uterus in position are**
   a) the cardinal or lateral ligament ____
   b) the round ligaments of the uterus ____
   c) the broad ligament ____
   d) the suspensory ligament ____
   e) the levator ani muscle ____

3. **Concerning the uterus:**
   a) the uterovesical pouch separates the supravaginal cervix from the bladder ____
   b) the pouch of Douglas (rectouterine pouch) with the coils of intestines lie posteriorly ____
   c) the ureter lies 12 mm lateral to the supravaginal cervix ____
   d) the cervix is smaller than the body throughout life ____
   e) all sensory innervation is by fibres accompanying the sympathetic nerves ____

The Reproductive System

1. a) **TRUE**
   b) **TRUE**
   c) **TRUE**
   d) **FALSE**   It has extravaginal and intravaginal parts.
   e) **FALSE**   The internal os is between the body and the cervix. The external os is the opening of the cervix into the vagina.

2. a) **TRUE**   It extends from the cervix to the side wall. It is also known as the Mackenrodt's ligament.
   b) **TRUE**   They extend from the junction of the uterus and the tube to the labia majora of the vulva. They pass through the inguinal canal.
   c) **FALSE**   This is a double layer of peritoneum lying lateral to the uterus. It is too thin to support the uterus.
   d) **FALSE**   This is a peritoneal fold lateral to the ovary.
   e) **TRUE**   Its pubovaginalis part (sphincter vaginae) winds around the vagina and the fibres are inserted into the perineal body. This forms an important support to the uterus.

3. a) **FALSE**   The supravaginal cervix is directly related to the bladder. The pouch is at a higher level.
   b) **TRUE**   This is the lowest part of the peritoneal cavity and it is about 5.5 cm above the anal margin.
   c) **TRUE**   At this level it lies below the uterine artery (water under the bridge). Knowledge of this fact is important in avoiding damage to the ureter while performing a hysterectomy.
   d) **FALSE**   In fetal life and in childhood the cervix is much larger than the body of the uterus.
   e) **FALSE**   Sensation from the cervix is transmitted by fibres accompanying the parasympathetic nerves (pelvic splanchnic nerves) going to the sacral part of the cord.

The Reproductive System

4. **With respect to the ovary:**
   a) the vein from the left passes to the inferior vena cava ____
   b) its artery also supplies the cervix ____
   c) it is smoother and larger than the testis ____
   d) it can cause irritation of the femoral nerve if inflamed ____
   e) lymphatics draining the ovary pass to the inguinal nodes ____

5. **Concerning the fallopian (uterine) tube:**
   a) the infundibulum is the most medial part ____
   b) the infundibulum has fimbriae and the osteum ____
   c) it lies in the free edge of the broad ligament ____
   d) it is wholly clothed in peritoneum ____
   e) it contributes to the communication between the peritoneal cavity and the exterior ____

6. **Concerning the vagina:**
   a) the posterior fornix is deeper than the anterior fornix ____
   b) the posterior wall is devoid of peritoneal lining ____
   c) it is lined by columnar epithelium ____
   d) there are no glands in its mucosa ____
   e) its blood supply is solely by the vaginal artery ____

7. **The following structures may be felt in a vaginal examination:**
   a) ovary ____
   b) uterine tube ____
   c) round ligament of the uterus ____
   d) uterosacral ligament ____
   e) a stone in the lower part of the ureter ____

The Reproductive System

4. a) **FALSE** It usually joins the left renal vein.
   b) **FALSE** The ovarian artery anastomoses with the uterine artery but its supply may not extend up to the cervix.
   c) **FALSE** The ovary is smaller than the testis. Its surface is not smooth after puberty because of degeneration of successive corpora lutea.
   d) **FALSE** The ovary lies on the obturator nerve and may cause pain along the medial part of the thigh, if inflamed.
   e) **FALSE** They follow the course of the blood vessels and drain to the para-aortic nodes.

5. a) **FALSE** It is the most lateral part of the tube.
   b) **TRUE**
   c) **TRUE** The broad ligament also carries the ovary, the uterine and ovarian vessels, nerves and lymphatics as well as the round ligament and the ovarian ligament.
   d) **FALSE** The interstitial part which pierces the uterine wall is not clothed in peritoneum.
   e) **TRUE** The osteum opens into the peritoneal cavity.

6. a) **TRUE**
   b) **FALSE** Peritoneum lines the upper part of the posterior wall and is reflected onto the rectum, forming the pouch of Douglas.
   c) **FALSE** It is lined by stratified squamous epithelium.
   d) **TRUE**
   e) **FALSE** There is a rich anastomosis on the vaginal wall between branches of the uterine, vaginal and internal pudendal arteries.

7. a) **TRUE**
   b) **TRUE**
   c) **FALSE**
   d) **TRUE**
   e) **TRUE** As the ureter lies close to the lateral fornix.

The Reproductive System

8. **The female breast lies on**
   a) pectoralis major
   b) pectoralis minor
   c) serratus anterior
   d) the upper part of the rectus sheath
   e) the upper six ribs

9. **Tumour cells from the breast may spread through lymphatics to**
   a) axillary lymph nodes
   b) parasternal (internal thoracic) nodes
   c) the opposite breast
   d) inguinal nodes
   e) the peritoneal cavity and liver

10. **With regard to the mammary gland in the female:**
    a) it is attached to the deep fascia
    b) it contains tubulo-alveolar glands which develop from ectoderm
    c) there is a considerable increase in alveoli (acini) at puberty
    d) its veins drain into intercostal veins
    e) the axillary tail may be deep to the deep fascia

11. **The scrotum**
    a) is supplied anteriorly by the ilioinguinal nerve
    b) is supplied posteriorly by branches of the pudendal nerve
    c) derives its blood supply entirely from branches of the internal pudendal artery
    d) has its dartos muscle deep to the deep fascia
    e) contains only the testes

The Reproductive System

8. a) **TRUE** The major part of the breast tissue lies on this muscle.
   b) **FALSE** This muscle lies deep to pectoralis major.
   c) **TRUE**
   d) **TRUE** Its lower medial edge lies on this.
   e) **FALSE** It lies on the second to sixth ribs. The first rib is under the clavicle.

9. a) **TRUE** 75% of lymph from the breast drains into this group of nodes.
   b) **TRUE** Especially from the medial part through the intercostal spaces.
   c) **TRUE** Especially when the normal channels are blocked.
   d) **TRUE** When the normal channels are blocked.
   e) **TRUE**

10. a) **FALSE** The glandular tissue has no attachment. The ligaments of Cooper extend from the deep fascia to the skin.
    b) **TRUE**
    c) **FALSE** An increase in alveoli occurs prior to lactation.
    d) **TRUE** Tumour cells can reach the vertebrae through this route.
    e) **TRUE** And it lies on the medial wall of the axilla.

11. a) **TRUE**
    b) **TRUE**
    c) **FALSE** The external pudendal artery (femoral) and the cremasteric artery (inferior epigastric) also supply the scrotum.
    d) **FALSE** The dartos muscle is in the superficial fascia. The scrotum does not have deep fascia.
    e) **FALSE** The scrotum contains the testes, epididymides, and the lower parts of the spermatic cords.

The Reproductive System

12. **Lymphatics from the testes drain into**
    a) the superficial inguinal nodes
    b) the deep inguinal nodes
    c) the common iliac nodes
    d) the external iliac nodes
    e) the para-aortic nodes

13. **The prostate gland**
    a) is homologous with the uterus
    b) contains no muscular fibres
    c) is surrounded by a venous plexus draining into the vertebral plexus
    d) has a median lobe palpable per rectum
    e) is traversed by the ductus deferens

14. **The ductus deferens**
    a) is approximately the same length as the thoracic duct
    b) has an ampulla at its commencement
    c) passes through the deep inguinal ring medial to the inferior epigastric artery
    d) lies medial to the seminal vesicle at the base of the bladder
    e) can be felt through the coverings of the spermatic cord because of its firm consistency

15. **Concerning the seminal vesicle:**
    a) it is normally felt by rectal examination
    b) it stores spermatozoa
    c) its secretion imparts motility to sperm
    d) it contracts by stimulation of the pelvic splanchnic nerves (parasympathetic)
    e) it has smooth muscle in its wall

The Reproductive System

12. a) **FALSE**
    b) **FALSE**
    c) **FALSE**
    d) **FALSE**
    e) **TRUE**

13. a) **FALSE**
    b) **FALSE** It has a fibromuscular stroma.
    c) **TRUE** Through this route tumour cells from the prostate can reach the vertebrae.
    d) **FALSE** Even when enlarged the median lobe is not palpable per rectum, as it extends forwards into the bladder. The lateral lobes, when enlarged, may be felt per rectum.
    e) **FALSE** It is traversed by the ejaculatory duct formed by the union of the ductus deferens and the duct of the seminal vesicle.

14. a) **TRUE** It is about 45 cm long, as are the spinal cord and the distance between the incisor teeth and the cardiac end of the stomach.
    b) **FALSE** It commences as the continuation of the tail of the epididymis. The ampulla is the dilation at its terminal part.
    c) **FALSE** The deep ring is lateral to the inferior epigastric artery.
    d) **TRUE**
    e) **TRUE**

15. a) **FALSE** It can be felt only when enlarged.
    b) **FALSE** The spermatozoa are stored in the epididymis and the ductus. However, the secretion of the seminal vesicles contributes about 80% of the volume of the seminal fluid (semen).
    c) **TRUE**
    d) **FALSE** Sympathetic stimulation produces contraction of the seminal vesicle during ejaculation.
    e) **TRUE**

339

The Reproductive System

16. Concerning the penis:

a) the bulb of the penis is part of the corpus cavernosum _____

b) the glans penis is the expanded distal end of the corpus spongiosum _____

c) the corpus spongiosum is traversed by the urethra _____

d) the bulbourethral glands open into the bulbar part of the penile urethra _____

e) all the lymph vessels drain primarily into the superficial inguinal nodes _____

The Reproductive System

16. a) **FALSE** The bulb is the proximal part of the corpus spongiosum.
    b) **TRUE**
    c) **TRUE**
    d) **TRUE**
    e) **FALSE** The glans penis drains primarily into the deep inguinal nodes.

The Reproductive System

Picture questions

Identify the numbered structures in the following illustrations from the choices given

Question 1

1. ____
2. ____
3. ____
4. ____
5. ____
6. ____
7. ____
8. ____

    A. Opening of bulbourethral gland
    B. Glans penis
    C. Membranous urethra
    D. Navicular fossa
    E. Urethral crest
    F. Prostatic urethra
    G. Penile urethra
    H. Colliculus seminalis

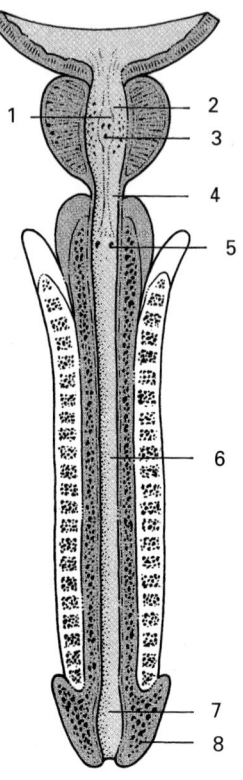

The Reproductive System

Question 2
1. ___
2. ___
3. ___
4. ___
5. ___
6. ___
7. ___
8. ___
9. ___
10. ___
11. ___
12. ___

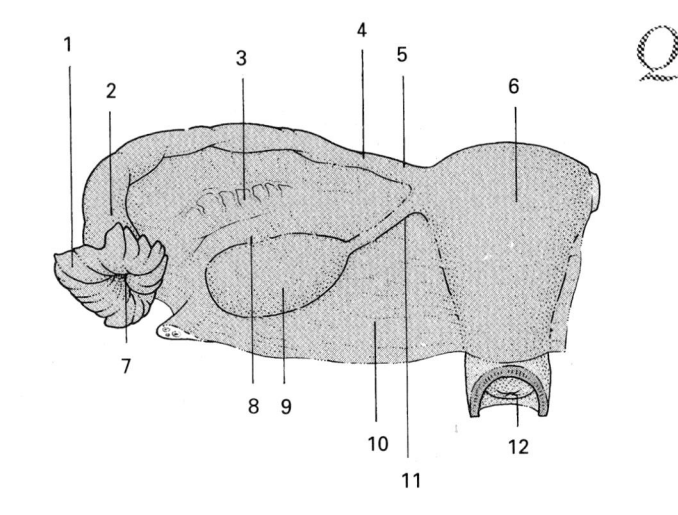

A. Epoophoron
B. Uterus
C. Ostium
D. Ovary
E. Fimbria
F. External os
G. Ampulla of uterine tube
H. Ligament of ovary
I. Broad ligament
J. Isthmus of uterine tube
K. Mesovarium
L. Infundibulum

Answers on page 346   343

The Reproductive System

Question 3
1. ___
2. ___
3. ___
4. ___
5. ___
6. ___
7. ___
8. ___

A. Ligament of ovary
B. Suspensory ligament of ovary
C. Ovary
D. Midline artery
E. Anastomoses between uterine and ovarian arteries
F. Ovarian artery
G. Uterine artery
H. Vaginal artery

Question 4
1. ___
2. ___
3. ___
4. ___
5. ___
6. ___
7. ___
8. ___

A. Internal os
B. Vestibule
C. Uterine tube
D. Fundus
E. Intramural part of uterine tube
F. Vagina
G. Cavity of body of uterus
H. External os

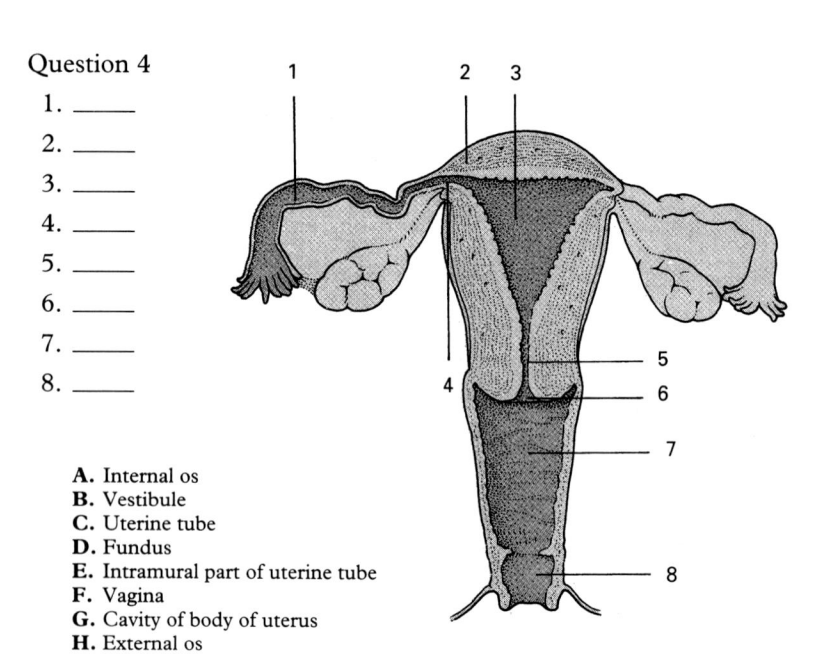

The Reproductive System

Question 5
1. ____
2. ____
3. ____
4. ____
5. ____
6. ____
7. ____

A. Ischiopubic ramus
B. Perineal membrane
C. Corpus spongiosum
D. Crus penis
E. Corpus cavernosum
F. Glans penis
G. Bulb of penis

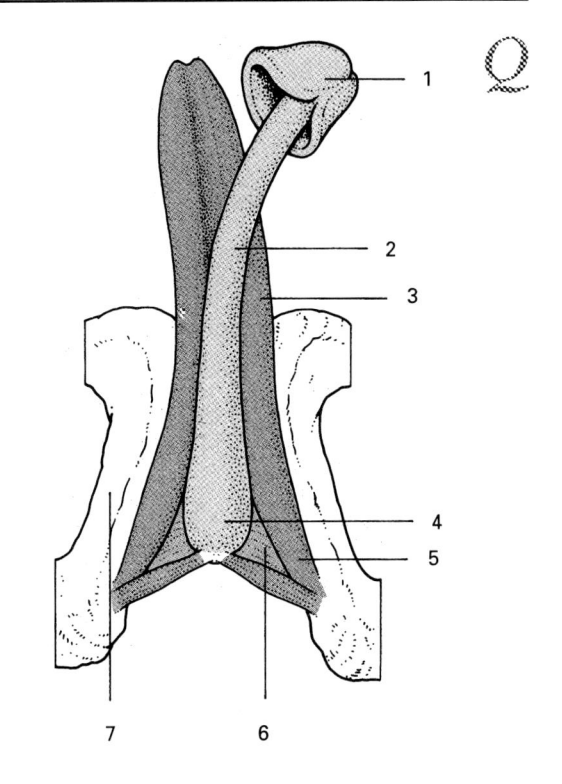

Answers on pages 346 and 347

The Reproductive System

A Picture questions

Question 1
1. **E** Urethral crest
2. **F** Prostatic urethra
3. **H** Colliculus seminalis
4. **C** Membranous urethra
5. **A** Opening of bulbourethral gland
6. **G** Penile urethra
7. **D** Navicular fossa
8. **B** Glans penis

Question 2
1. **E** Fimbria
2. **L** Infundibulum
3. **A** Epoophoron
4. **G** Ampulla of uterine tube
5. **J** Isthmus of uterine tube
6. **B** Uterus
7. **C** Ostium
8. **K** Mesovarium
9. **D** Ovary
10. **I** Broad ligament
11. **H** Ligament of ovary
12. **F** External os

Question 3
1. **F** Ovarian artery
2. **B** Suspensory ligament of ovary
3. **C** Ovary
4. **E** Anastomoses between uterine and ovarian arteries
5. **A** Ligament of ovary
6. **G** Uterine artery
7. **H** Vaginal artery
8. **D** Midline artery

The Reproductive System

Question 4
1. **C** Uterine tube
2. **D** Fundus
3. **G** Cavity of body of uterus
4. **E** Intramural part of uterine tube
5. **A** Internal os
6. **H** External os
7. **F** Vagina
8. **B** Vestibule

Question 5
1. **F** Glans penis
2. **C** Corpus spongiosum
3. **E** Corpus cavernosum
4. **G** Bulb of penis
5. **D** Crus penis
6. **B** Perineal membrane
7. **A** Ischiopubic ramus

The Reproductive System

Clinical problems

1. Prolapse of the uterus into the vagina is a frequently encountered gynaecological condition. With advancing age there is increased relaxation and loss of tone of the muscular and ligamentous structures that support the uterus. The condition is more common in women who have had multiple childbirths, as lacerations and overstretching of the supporting tissues during childbirth greatly enhance the chances of prolapse. What is the normal position of the uterus? What do the terms 'anteflexion' and 'anteversion' indicate? Does the position of the uterus normally change? What are the main structures supporting the uterus?

2. Epidural anaesthesia is often given to relieve pain during childbirth. Which nerves transmit pain from the uterus and cervix?

Answers on page 350

The Reproductive System

A Clinical problems

1. In prolapse of the uterus, the uterus descends into the vagina and the cervix may be seen near the vestibule or even outside on straining. When the bladder is empty a normal uterus is bent forward on the vagina (anteverted), and the angle between the long axes of the two is open anteriorly and a little over 90°. In addition, the uterus is anteflexed, which denotes the anteriorly open angle between the body and the cervix. The uterus is normally a mobile organ. When the bladder fills, the uterus is elevated from its anteverted position and may even be retroverted (opposite of anteversion) by the upper border of the bladder. When the bladder empties it returns to its original position. The principal support of the uterus is the pelvic diaphragm formed by the levator ani muscle. Posteriorly, the diaphragm is closed by the anococcygeal raphe; in between the vagina and the rectum it is anchored onto, and reinforced by, the perineal body. In front of the vagina the gap between the two levator ani is closed by the urogenital diaphragm. Besides the pelvic diaphragm, the uterus is also supported by the lateral cervical ligaments (cardinal or Mackenrodt's ligaments) and the uterosacral ligaments. These are condensations of parametrial connective tissue at the base of the broad ligament. The ureters are closely related to the cardinal ligaments and are vulnerable in hysterectomy and repair of prolapse. The ureter crosses below the uterine artery ('water under the bridge').

2. Pain from the body of the uterus is transmitted by the afferents accompanying the sympathetic nerves. These then reach the spinal cord by passing through the hypogastric and aortic plexuses, splanchnic nerves, and sympathetic chain, and from this through the white rami communicantes to the spinal cord. Blockage of nerve roots up to the level of T10 will relieve the uterine pain. Pain from the cervix is transmitted by the afferents accompanying the pelvic splanchnic nerves to the S2–S4 segments of the cord.

The Reproductive System

3. A 35-year-old man complaining of a scrotal swelling was seen by his doctor. On palpation the testis was found to be enlarged and a tumour of the testis was suspected. What structures are normally felt on examination of the scrotum? How are these distinguished from one another? Testicular tumours spread through the lymphatics. Which lymph node groups will be examined for possible metastases?

4. A 32-year-old school teacher consulted a surgeon about a vasectomy. His wife had had three caesarean sections already and they had decided not to have any more children. Vasectomy involves ligation and cutting of the ductus deferens. For sterilisation it is done on both sides. The ductus lies in the spermatic cord. What are the constituents of the cord and what are the characteristic features of the ductus deferens?

The Reproductive System

3. The testes, epididymides and spermatic cords lie in the scrotum and can be felt on palpation. The testis is smooth and round and can easily be felt in the scrotum. The epididymis is felt along the posterior aspect of the testis, and the spermatic cord in the upper part of the scrotum. The ductus deferens is felt as a firm tube inside the spermatic cord. Lymph from the testis drains into the para-aortic lymph nodes (not the inguinal) and when enlarged these may be palpable on deep palpation of the abdomen. Further spread may involve the mediastinal and supraclavicular nodes.

4. For vasectomy, a skin incision is made at the root of the scrotum under local anaesthesia and the ductus deferens is identified among the constituents of the spermatic cord. The ductus has a hard, whip-cord-like feel because of the muscle layers in its wall. The components of the spermatic cord are the ductus with its artery, the testicular artery, and the nerves accompanying it, the pampiniform plexus of veins, lymph vessels and the remnant of the processus vaginalis. All these are covered by the internal spermatic fascia (derived from the transversalis fascia), the cremasteric muscle and fascia (internal oblique) and the external spermatic fascia (external oblique).

The Reproductive System

5. A 52-year-old woman who noticed a swelling in her breast was seen by a surgeon. On examination a lump was detected in the outer quadrant of the right breast. Skin over the lump was dimpled and the right nipple was retracted. The swelling in the breast was not fixed to the underlying muscles. However, examination of the axilla revealed enlargement of the lymph nodes. An initial diagnosis of cancer of the breast was made which was confirmed by biopsy. She was treated by removal of her right breast (simple mastectomy) and removal of the lymph nodes in the axilla. This was followed by radiotherapy.

   What caused dimpling of the skin over the tumour and the retraction of the nipple? Which muscles lie deep to the breast? Which lymph nodes drain the breast? Which nerves are vulnerable in dissection of the axilla for removal of lymph nodes? What would be the effect of damage to these nerves?

The Reproductive System

5. The breast overlies pectoralis major and serratus anterior and, in the lower medial part, the rectus sheath. The breast lies in the superficial fascia and is not attached to the underlying muscles or their fascial covering. Dimpling of the skin over the tumour is caused by infiltration of the tumour into the ligaments of Cooper, which are fibrous septa connecting the skin and the underlying deep fascia. Retraction of the nipple is due to contraction of the ducts caused by the tumour.

   The breast is drained by the axillary lymph nodes as well as the lymph nodes along the internal thoracic artery. The axillary lymph nodes are divided into five groups — the anterior or pectoral along the lower border of the pectoralis minor, the posterior or subscapular along the subscapular vessels, the lateral or brachial along the lower part of the axillary vein, the central in the fat in the axilla, and the apical at the apex of the axilla. Two nerves are vulnerable in the operation of axillary clearance: the long thoracic nerve, which supplies the serratus anterior, and the thoracodorsal nerve supplying the latissimus dorsi. Paralysis of serratus anterior results in winging of the scapula, where the medial border of the scapula becomes more prominent on protraction. Every effort should be made to avoid cutting these nerves.

The Endocrine System

The Endocrine System

THE ENDOCRINE GLANDS

True/False

1. **The pituitary gland**
   a) is connected to the hypothalamus
   b) has a posterior lobe derived from endoderm
   c) lies inferior to the optic chiasma
   d) lies superior to the sphenoid sinus
   e) receives its entire blood supply from branches of the internal carotid artery

2. **With regard to the pituitary gland:**
   a) the anterior lobe is developed from the Rathke's pouch of the buccal cavity
   b) hormones from the hypothalamus are transported to the anterior lobe through neurones
   c) hormones from the hypothalamus are transported to the posterior pituitary through neurones
   d) a growth hormone is produced by the anterior lobe
   e) a pituitary tumour may produce bitemporal hemianopia

3. **Concerning the thyroid gland:**
   a) all the veins drain into the internal jugular vein
   b) the arterial supply is entirely from branches of the external carotid and subclavian arteries
   c) the isthmus lies in front of the second and third tracheal rings
   d) it is enclosed in the pretracheal fascia
   e) it moves with deglutition

The Endocrine System

THE ENDOCRINE GLANDS

1. a) **TRUE**   The infundibulum connects it to the hypothalamus.
   b) **FALSE**   The posterior lobe is derived from the diencephalon.
   c) **TRUE**   The two are separated by the diaphragma sellae.
   d) **TRUE**   The pituitary can be surgically approached through the sphenoid sinus.
   e) **FALSE**   It also receives blood from the posterior cerebral artery (basilar, vertebral).

2. a) **TRUE**
   b) **FALSE**   They pass to the anterior lobe via the hypothalamo-hypophyseal portal system of veins.
   c) **TRUE**
   d) **TRUE**
   e) **TRUE**   By compressing the optic chiasma.

3. a) **FALSE**   The superior and middle thyroid veins drain into the internal jugular; the inferior thyroid veins drain into the left brachiocephalic vein.
   b) **FALSE**   There is usually a thyroidea ima artery which is a branch of the brachiocephalic artery or the arch of the aorta.
   c) **TRUE**
   d) **TRUE**   The fascia splits to form the capsule.
   e) **TRUE**   As the pretracheal fascia is attached to the thyroid cartilage.

The Endocrine System

4. **The following statements about the thyroid gland are true:**
   a) it is derived from the third branchial arch
   b) the ultimobranchial body provides some cells
   c) thyroxine is the only hormone produced
   d) it may be abnormally present at the back of the tongue
   e) the recurrent laryngeal nerve is vulnerable in thyroid surgery

5. **Regarding the parathyroid glands:**
   a) there are always four glands
   b) they are closely related to the thyroid gland
   c) they may be abnormally present in the mediastinum
   d) the inferior gland develops from the fourth pharyngeal pouch along with the thymus
   e) removal produces tetany due to lowered serum calcium

6. **The right adrenal gland**
   a) is a direct posterior relation of the inferior vena cava
   b) is related to the bare area of the liver
   c) receives blood from the inferior phrenic artery
   d) drains to the renal vein
   e) is closely related to the right coeliac ganglion

7. **Concerning the adrenal glands:**
   a) they receive postganglionic fibres from the greater splanchnic nerves
   b) each gland has one artery, and three veins draining it
   c) they receive blood from the renal arteries
   d) the medulla is developed from neuroectoderm
   e) each gland lies inside the respective renal capsule

The Endocrine System

4. a) **FALSE** It is mostly derived from the thyroglossal duct.
    b) **TRUE** The C cells are derived from this.
    c) **FALSE** The thyroid also produces triiodothyronine and thyrocalcitonin.
    d) **TRUE** A lingual thyroid may occur as the thyroglossal duct commences at the foramen caecum of the tongue.
    e) **TRUE** The nerve crosses the inferior thyroid artery near the lower pole of the gland.

5. a) **FALSE** There are usually four — two superior and two inferior — but the number is variable.
    b) **TRUE** Towards its posterior aspect.
    c) **TRUE** As aberrant parathyroid.
    d) **FALSE** The inferior glands and the thymus are derived from the third pouch, and the superior gland from the fourth.
    e) **TRUE**

6. a) **TRUE**
    b) **TRUE**
    c) **TRUE**
    d) **FALSE** It drains to the inferior vena cava.
    e) **TRUE**

7. a) **FALSE** It is preganglionic fibres in the greater splanchnic nerves that end in the adrenal medulla.
    b) **FALSE** Each gland has three arteries and one vein.
    c) **TRUE** The renal artery is one of the three arteries supplying the gland; the others being branches from the inferior phrenic artery and abdominal aorta.
    d) **TRUE**
    e) **TRUE**

The Endocrine System

8. **Concerning the left adrenal gland:**
   a) it is crossed posteriorly by the pancreas
   b) it receives blood from the aorta
   c) the left adrenal vein is longer than the right
   d) it is closely related to the spleen
   e) it lies behind the stomach

The Endocrine System

8. a) **FALSE** The pancreas crosses in front.
   b) **TRUE** Both glands receive branches from the aorta.
   c) **TRUE** The left adrenal vein joins the renal vein, whereas the right drains to the inferior vena cava.
   d) **TRUE**
   e) **TRUE** It is separated from it by the lesser sac.

The Endocrine System

Picture questions

Identify the numbered structures in the following illustrations from the choices given

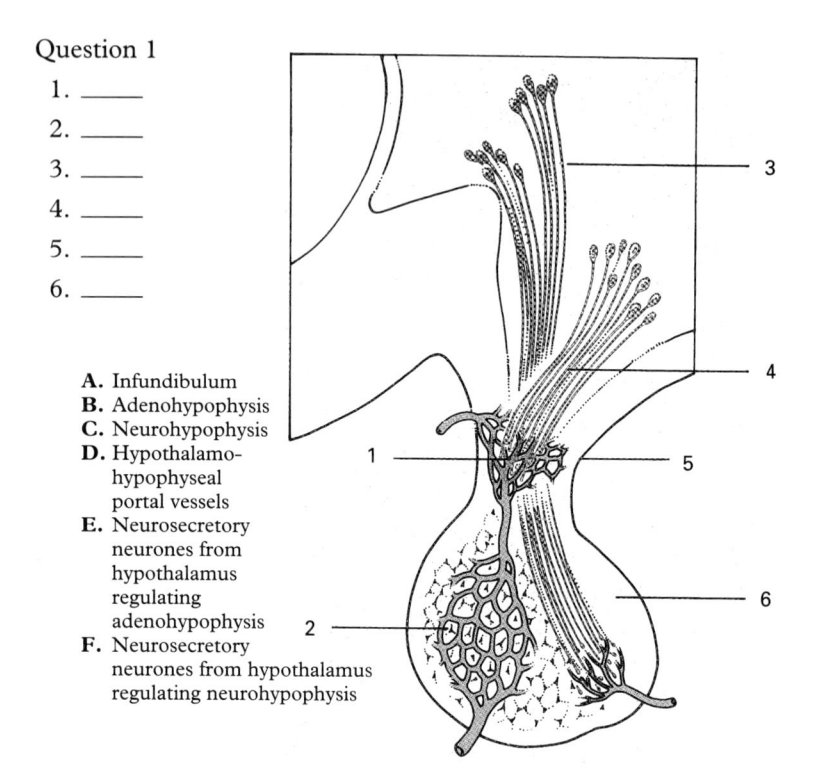

Question 1

1. ____
2. ____
3. ____
4. ____
5. ____
6. ____

A. Infundibulum
B. Adenohypophysis
C. Neurohypophysis
D. Hypothalamo-hypophyseal portal vessels
E. Neurosecretory neurones from hypothalamus regulating adenohypophysis
F. Neurosecretory neurones from hypothalamus regulating neurohypophysis

The Endocrine System

Question 2
1. ____
2. ____
3. ____
4. ____
5. ____
6. ____

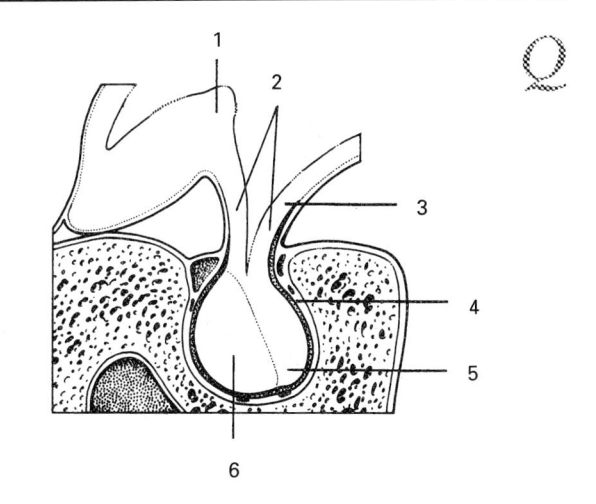

A. Hypophyseal (pituitary) fossa
B. Neurohypophysis
C. Hypothalamus
D. Adenohypophysis
E. Infundibular stem
F. Pars tuberalis

Question 3
1. ____
2. ____
3. ____
4. ____
5. ____
6. ____
7. ____
8. ____
9. ____
10. ____
11. ____

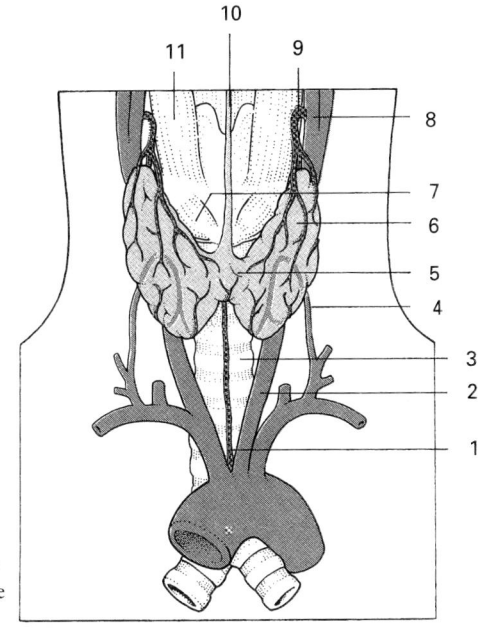

A. Trachea
B. Left common carotid artery
C. Levator glandulae thyroidiae
D. Cricothyroid muscle
E. Thyroidea ima artery
F. Lateral lobe of thyroid gland
G. Superior thyroid artery
H. Thyrohyoid muscle
I. Inferior thyroid artery
J. External carotid artery
K. Isthmus of thyroid gland

Answers on page 366

The Endocrine System

Question 4
1. ___
2. ___
3. ___
4. ___
5. ___
6. ___
7. ___
8. ___
9. ___
10. ___
11. ___
12. ___
13. ___

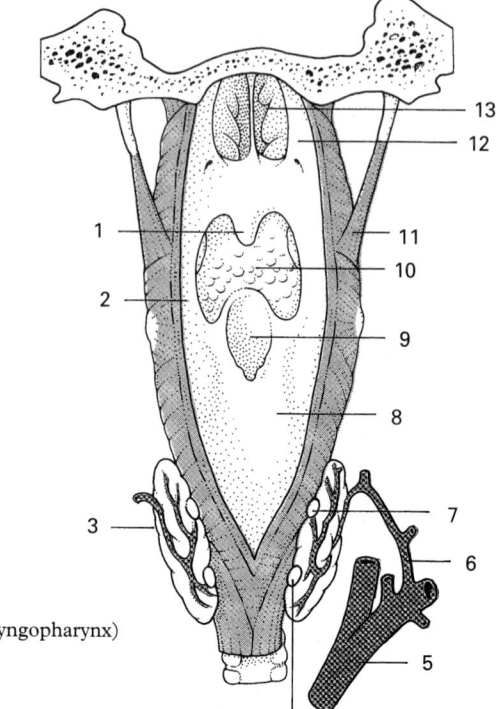

A. Nasal cavity
B. Inlet of larynx
C. Hypopharynx (laryngopharynx)
D. Subclavian artery
E. Uvula
F. Nasopharynx
G. Oral cavity
H. Superior parathyroid
I. Inferior parathyroid
J. Oropharynx
K. Stylopharyngeus muscle
L. Inferior thyroid artery
M. Thyroid gland

The Endocrine System

Question 5

1. ____
2. ____
3. ____
4. ____
5. ____
6. ____
7. ____
8. ____
9. ____
10. ____

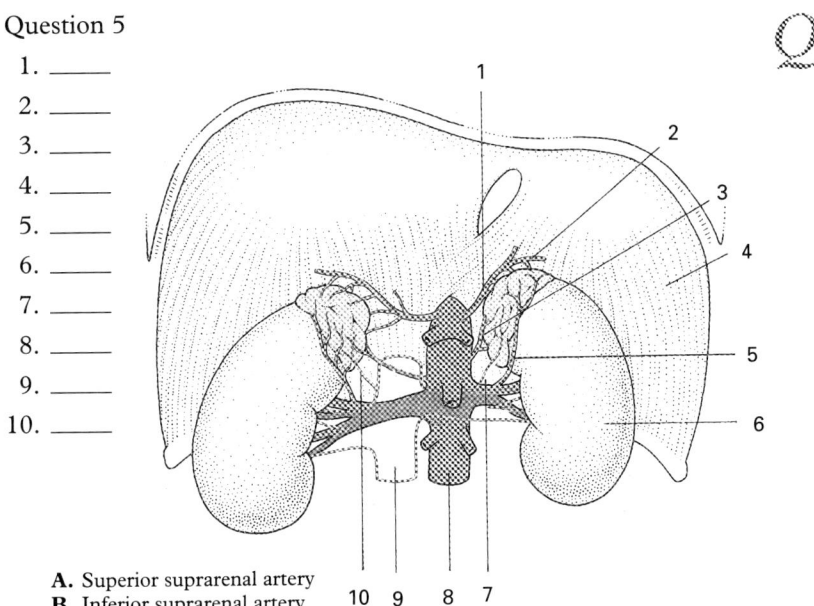

A. Superior suprarenal artery
B. Inferior suprarenal artery
C. Inferior vena cava
D. Inferior phrenic artery
E. Right suprarenal vein to join inferior vena cava
F. Middle suprarenal artery
G. Left kidney
H. Left suprarenal vein to join left renal vein
I. Diaphragm
J. Aorta

Answers on page 367

The Endocrine System

A Picture questions

Question 1
1. **D** Hypothalamo-hypophyseal portal vessels
2. **B** Adenohypophysis
3. **F** Neurosecretory neurones from hypothalamus regulating neurohypophysis
4. **E** Neurosecretory neurones from hypothalamus regulating adenohypophysis
5. **A** Infundibulum
6. **C** Neurohypophysis

Question 2
1. **C** Hypothalamus
2. **E** Infundibular stem
3. **F** Pars tuberalis
4. **A** Hypophyseal (pituitary) fossa
5. **B** Neurohypophysis
6. **D** Adenohypophysis

Question 3
1. **E** Thyroidea ima artery
2. **B** Left common carotid artery
3. **A** Trachea
4. **I** Inferior thyroid artery
5. **K** Isthmus of thyroid gland
6. **F** Lateral lobe of thyroid gland
7. **D** Cricothyroid muscle
8. **J** External carotid artery
9. **G** Superior thyroid artery
10. **C** Levator glandulae thyroidiae
11. **H** Thyrohyoid muscle

The Endocrine System

Question 4
1. **E** Uvula
2. **J** Oropharynx
3. **M** Thyroid gland
4. **I** Inferior parathyroid
5. **D** Subclavian artery
6. **L** Inferior thyroid artery
7. **H** Superior parathyroid
8. **C** Hypopharynx (laryngopharynx)
9. **B** Inlet of larynx
10. **G** Oral cavity
11. **K** Stylopharyngeus muscle
12. **F** Nasopharynx
13. **A** Nasal cavity

Question 5
1. **D** Inferior phrenic artery
2. **A** Superior suprarenal artery
3. **F** Middle suprarenal artery
4. **I** Diaphragm
5. **B** Inferior suprarenal artery
6. **G** Left kidney
7. **H** Left suprarenal vein to join left renal vein
8. **J** Aorta
9. **C** Inferior vena cava
10. **E** Right suprarenal vein to join inferior vena cava

The Endocrine System

Clinical problems

1. A 35-year-old woman was admitted to hospital complaining of severe headache and amenorrhoea. She also complains of weakness, lethargy and general slowing of her reactions. X-ray of the skull showed enlargement of the sella turcica, separation of the anterior clinoid processes and thinning of the posterior clinoids. Further tests revealed a chromophobe adenoma of the pituitary gland inhibiting thyroid functions and sex functions. As the patient was waiting for surgery, her headache became less. However, she started to have problems with her vision and on testing was found to have developed bitemporal hemianopia. From your knowledge of anatomy can you explain the signs and symptoms this patient had?

2. A patient having a rounded swelling at the back of the tongue was diagnosed as having a lingual thyroid. What is the embryological explanation of this condition? What is a thyroglossal cyst? In what other unusual site might one encounter thyroid tissue?

The Endocrine System

A Clinical problems

1. A chromophobe adenoma is a common pituitary tumour. As the tumour grows it expands the sella turcica. Pressure on the diaphragma sellae causes severe headache. The chromophobe cells possess no active secretion of their own, but the tumour compresses the acidophil and basophil cells. These cells produce trophic hormones which regulate the functions of the thyroid gland and adrenal cortex as well as the gonads (producing sex steroids). Levels of TSH, ACTH and gonadotrophic hormones are therefore reduced, producing amenorrhoea and signs of hypothyroidism.

    As the tumour grows further, it breaks through the diaphragma sellae and the headache diminishes. However, at this stage it will compress the optic chiasma lying just above the pituitary gland and produce the characteristic bitemporal hemianopia.

2. The thyroid develops from the thyroglossal duct. This starts from the region of the foramen caecum of the tongue. The duct descends through the floor of the mouth in intimate contact with the hyoid, and expands to form the thyroid gland in the region of the thyroid cartilage. The gland usually loses its connection to the foramen caecum. If the whole or part of the duct remains patent it will give rise to a thyroglossal cyst. In this condition, as the duct is adherent to the hyoid bone, dissection of its tract and its removal may require cutting the body of the hyoid bone. Rarely, the whole or part of the thyroglossal duct develops as the gland in the region of the foramen caecum (as in this case), giving rise to a lingual thyroid. The duct may descend beyond its normal position into the mediastinum giving rise to a mediastinal thyroid. Enlargement of a mediastinal thyroid will produce a mediastinal goitre, causing pressure symptoms on adjoining structures.

The Endocrine System

3. A patient who was investigated for a swelling in the neck and change in the voice was found to have a malignant tumour of the thyroid gland. She had slight drooping of the eyelid and noticed dryness of the skin of her face on the side of the swelling. What are the characteristics of an enlarged thyroid? Can you explain this patient's signs and symptoms? Which muscles need to be cut to expose the gland? Which vessels are ligated and cut before the gland is removed? Which nerves are at risk in thyroidectomy?

4. A patient may develop signs of hypoparathyroidism after thyroidectomy. Why? What are the signs of hypoparathyroidism? Where are the parathyroid glands located?

The Endocrine System

3. As the thyroid gland is enclosed in the pretracheal fascia it moves with deglutition. A swelling in the neck which moves on swallowing invariably has its origin in the thyroid. A malignant tumour may spread into the adjoining structures. It may erode the trachea, oesophagus or even the carotid sheath. Involvement of the recurrent laryngeal nerve may cause a change in the voice. Involvement of the sympathetic trunk causes Horner's syndrome, characterised by slight drooping of the eyelid, meiosis, and anhydrosis on the same side of the face.

   The infrahyoid muscles cover the thyroid gland. If these need to be cut to obtain a good exposure, they are severed at their upper ends as the nerves (ansa cervicalis) enter the lower part. The thyroid gland is supplied by three arteries — the superior and inferior thyroid arteries and, occasionally, the thyroidea ima. It is drained by three veins — the superior, middle and inferior thyroid veins. The superior laryngeal and recurrent laryngeal nerves, which cross the superior and inferior thyroid arteries respectively, are at risk in thyroid surgery.

4. Loss of parathyroid gland function will reduce the blood calcium level and produce tetany. This is manifested as tingling and numbness in the face, fingers and toes, followed by spasm of various muscle groups. The symptoms will be relieved by intravenous administration of calcium gluconate. The parathyroids are closely related to the thyroid gland and are at risk in thyroidectomy. There are four glands: an upper and a lower pair. Each gland has an oval shape, is about 1 cm in size and is yellowish-brown in colour. The upper pair is found on the posterolateral border of the thyroid immediately above the point of entry of the inferior thyroid artery. The lower pair is more variable in position and may be found at the lower pole of the thyroid or anywhere down the line to the upper pole of the thymus. The lower parathyroids develop with the thymus, hence the variation in location.

The Lymphatic System

The Lymphatic System

THE LYMPHATIC SYSTEM

True/False

1. **The cysterna chyli**
   a) is a dilated lymph sac
   b) lies in the posterior mediastinum
   c) receives lymph from the abdomen and thorax
   d) is closely related to the aorta
   e) continues upwards as the thoracic duct

2. **The thoracic duct**
   a) enters the thorax through the caval opening in the diaphragm
   b) has the aorta on its right
   c) in the lower part of the thorax, lies to the right of the oesophagus
   d) lies posterior to the left carotid sheath in the neck
   e) terminates at the junction of the left subclavian and internal jugular veins

3. **The thoracic duct**
   a) lies to the right of the oesophagus at the thoracic inlet
   b) lies to the left of the azygos vein
   c) is closely related to the thoracic vertebrae
   d) receives lymph from the thorax
   e) receives lymph from the entire body except the right side of the thorax, the head and neck and the right upper limb

4. **The superficial inguinal lymph nodes receive lymph from**
   a) the skin above the umbilicus
   b) the great toe
   c) the little toe
   d) the anal canal
   e) the testes

The Lymphatic System

1. a) **TRUE**
   b) **FALSE** It lies in front of the first lumbar vertebra in the abdomen.
   c) **FALSE** It receives lymph from the entire abdomen and both lower limbs.
   d) **TRUE** It lies immediately to the right of the abdominal aorta.
   e) **TRUE**

2. a) **FALSE** It enters the thorax through the aortic orifice.
   b) **FALSE** The aorta lies to the left of the thoracic duct.
   c) **TRUE** It crosses to the left border at the level of T4 and ascends on the left border in the upper part.
   d) **TRUE** It curves laterally behind the carotid sheath.
   e) **TRUE**

3. a) **FALSE**
   b) **TRUE**
   c) **TRUE** It lies on the vertebrae in the lower part and may be torn in fractures of the vertebrae.
   d) **TRUE** The left bronchomediastinal trunk drains into it.
   e) **TRUE** The right bronchomediastinal trunk, right subclavian (from the upper limb) and right jugular trunk may join the great veins at the root of the neck directly.

4. a) **FALSE** From the skin below the umbilicus.
   b) **TRUE** The lymph vessels accompany the great saphenous vein.
   c) **FALSE** The lymph vessels of the little toe accompany the short saphenous vein and drain into the popliteal nodes and the deep inguinal nodes.
   d) **TRUE** The lower part of the anal canal drains into the superficial inguinal nodes.
   e) **FALSE** These drain into the para-aortic nodes.

The Lymphatic System

5. **The deep inguinal nodes**
   a) are usually about 10 in number
   b) lie lateral to the femoral vein
   c) drain the scrotum
   d) drain the glans penis in the male
   e) drain the uterus in the female

6. **Concerning the axillary lymph nodes:**
   a) they are arranged in five groups
   b) they drain lymph from the abdominal wall above the umbilicus
   c) they drain lymph from the breast
   d) the pectoral (anterior) group lies along the lower border of pectoralis major
   e) the lateral group drains the thumb

7. **Concerning the lymph nodes of the neck:**
   a) the superficial cervical nodes lie along the external jugular vein
   b) the deep cervical nodes lie along the internal jugular vein
   c) all the lymph from the tongue drains into the submandibular nodes
   d) the submandibular nodes lie deep to the submandibular gland
   e) the thyroid gland drains into the deep cervical nodes

8. **With regard to the spleen:**
   a) it can normally be felt at the costal margin
   b) accessory spleen may occur normally
   c) it is related to the left costodiaphragmatic recess
   d) the tail of the pancreas is related to the hilum
   e) its long axis is along the ninth rib

The Lymphatic System

5. a) **FALSE** There are usually about three nodes.
   b) **FALSE** They lie medial to the femoral vein in the femoral canal.
   c) **FALSE** The scrotum drains into the superficial inguinal nodes.
   d) **TRUE**
   e) **FALSE** Some lymphatics drain via the round ligament to the superficial inguinal nodes.

6. a) **TRUE** These are the anterior, posterior, lateral, central and apical groups.
   b) **TRUE**
   c) **TRUE** This is the major lymph node group draining the breast.
   d) **FALSE** This group lies deep to pectoralis major along the lower border of pectoralis minor.
   e) **TRUE** The upper limb drains into the lateral group.

7. a) **TRUE** They are in the posterior triangle and are closely related to the accessory nerve.
   b) **TRUE**
   c) **FALSE** The tongue also drains directly into the submental and deep cervical nodes.
   d) **FALSE** They lie superficial to the salivary gland.
   e) **TRUE**

8. a) **FALSE** It has to enlarge to twice its normal size before it is palpable.
   b) **TRUE** It is found commonly at the hilum. If left behind after splenectomy, the symptoms for which splenectomy was performed may persist.
   c) **TRUE** It is separated from the pleural cavity by the diaphragm.
   d) **TRUE** The pancreas can be damaged in splenectomy.
   e) **FALSE** The long axis of the spleen is along the tenth rib.

The Lymphatic System

9. **The following statements about the thymus are true:**
   a) it lies in the anterior mediastinum
   b) it is most prominent in children
   c) it lies in front of the pretracheal fascia
   d) it is derived from the fourth pharyngeal pouch, along with the inferior parathyroid gland
   e) T-lymphocytes are derived from it

9. a) **TRUE** It also extends into the superior mediastinum.
   b) **TRUE** After puberty the thymus starts to atrophy.
   c) **FALSE** It lies behind the pretracheal fascia.
   d) **FALSE** It is derived from the third pharyngeal pouch, along with the inferior parathyroid.
   e) **FALSE** T-lymphocytes differentiate in the thymus. They are derived from the bone marrow.

The Lymphatic System

Picture questions

Identify the numbered structures in the following illustrations from the choices given

Question 1
1. ___
2. ___
3. ___
4. ___
5. ___
6. ___
7. ___
8. ___
9. ___
10. ___
11. ___
12. ___

A. Aorta
B. Left brachiocephalic vein
C. Right lymph duct
D. Bronchomediastinal trunks
E. Left internal carotid artery
F. Oesophagus
G. Left subclavian vein
H. Jugular lymph trunk
I. Thoracic duct
J. Cisterna chyli
K. Subclavian lymph trunk
L. Left internal jugular vein

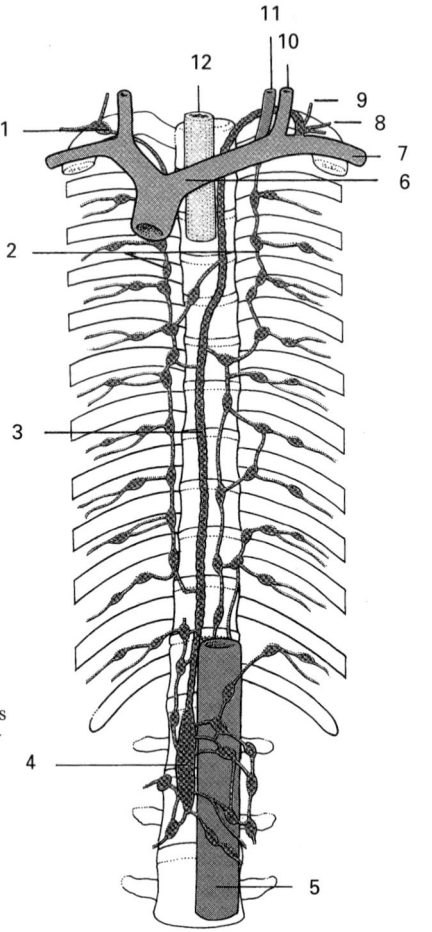

The Lymphatic System

Question 2
1. ____
2. ____
3. ____
4. ____
5. ____
6. ____
7. ____
8. ____
9. ____
10. ____
11. ____
12. ____
13. ____

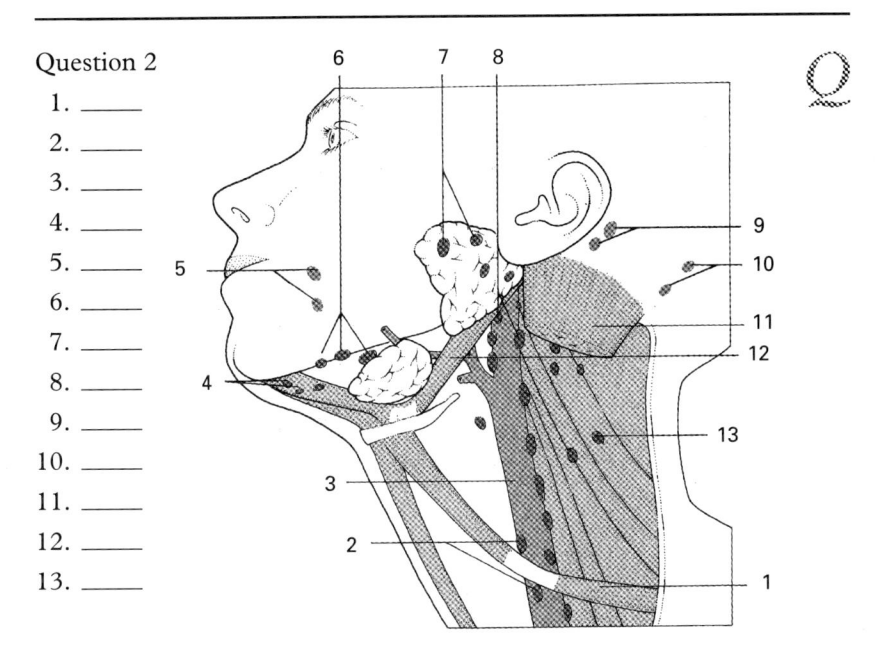

A. Omohyoid muscle
B. Submental nodes
C. Parotid nodes
D. Posterior auricular nodes
E. Occipital nodes
F. Superior cervical nodes
G. Inferior deep cervical nodes
H. Buccal nodes
I. Posterior belly of digastric muscle
J. Internal jugular vein
K. Submandibular nodes
L. Superior deep cervical nodes
M. Sternocleidomastoid muscle

Answers on page 384 381

The Lymphatic System

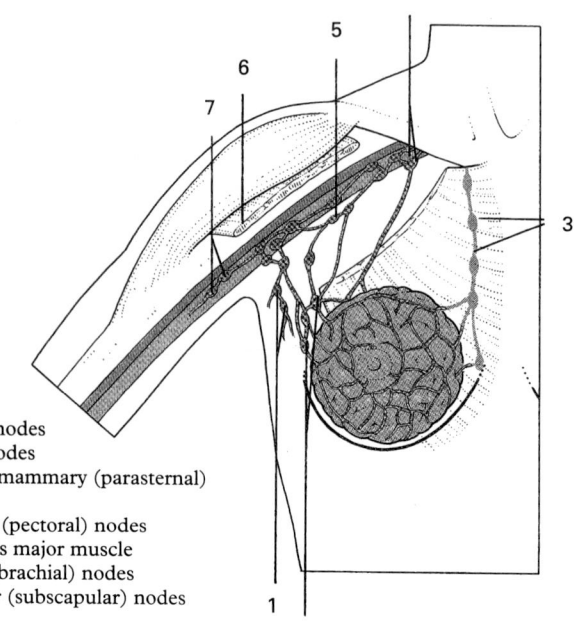

Question 3
1. ___
2. ___
3. ___
4. ___
5. ___
6. ___
7. ___

A. Central nodes
B. Apical nodes
C. Internal mammary (parasternal) nodes
D. Anterior (pectoral) nodes
E. Pectoralis major muscle
F. Lateral (brachial) nodes
G. Posterior (subscapular) nodes

Question 4
1. ___
2. ___
3. ___
4. ___
5. ___
6. ___
7. ___

A. Arch of aorta
B. Tracheobronchial nodes
C. Pulmonary nodes
D. Bronchomediastinal trunks
E. Trachea
F. Hilar lymph nodes
G. Oesophagus

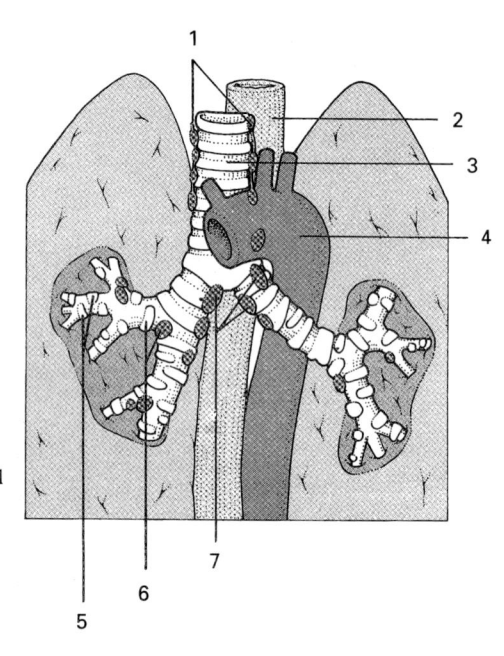

The Lymphatic System

Question 5

1. ____
2. ____
3. ____
4. ____
5. ____
6. ____
7. ____

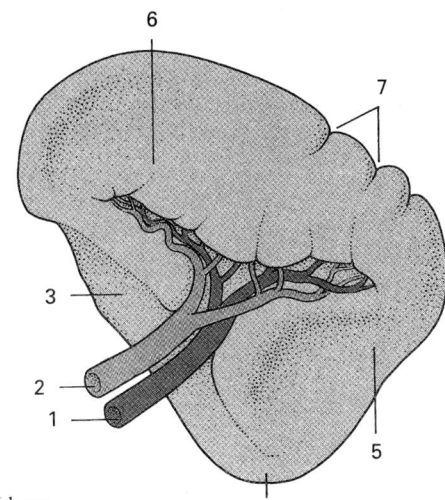

A. Splenic vein
B. Splenic artery
C. Surface related to left kidney
D. Splenic notches
E. Surface related to stomach
F. Surface related to colon
G. Inferior pole

Answers on pages 384 and 385

The Lymphatic System

A Picture questions

Question 1
1. C Right lymph duct
2. D Bronchomediastinal trunks
3. I Thoracic duct
4. J Cisterna chyli
5. A Aorta
6. B Left brachiocephalic vein
7. G Left subclavian vein
8. K Subclavian lymph trunk
9. H Jugular lymph trunk
10. L Left internal jugular vein
11. E Left common carotid artery
12. F Oesophagus

Question 2
1. A Omohyoid muscle
2. G Inferior deep cervical nodes
3. J Internal jugular vein
4. B Submental nodes
5. H Buccal nodes
6. K Submandibular nodes
7. C Parotid nodes
8. L Superior deep cervical nodes
9. D Posterior auricular nodes
10. E Occipital nodes
11. M Sternocleidomastoid muscle
12. I Posterior belly of digastric muscle
13. F Superior cervical nodes

Question 3
1. G Posterior (subscapular) nodes
2. D Anterior (pectoral) nodes
3. C Internal mammary (parasternal) nodes
4. B Apical nodes
5. A Central nodes
6. E Pectoralis major muscle
7. F Lateral (brachial) nodes

The Lymphatic System

Question 4
1. **D** Bronchomediastinal trunks
2. **G** Oesophagus
3. **E** Trachea
4. **A** Arch of aorta
5. **C** Pulmonary nodes
6. **F** Hilar lymph nodes
7. **B** Tracheobronchial nodes

Question 5
1. **A** Splenic vein
2. **B** Splenic artery
3. **C** Surface related to left kidney
4. **G** Inferior pole
5. **F** Surface related to colon
6. **E** Surface related to stomach
7. **D** Splenic notches

The Lymphatic System

Clinical problems

1. A patient presents with enlarged lymph nodes in the neck which are indurated (firm-to-hard in consistency). The physician suspects secondary malignancy and examines for the sites of the primary tumour. Where will he search for the primary growth?

2. Hodgkin's disease is a malignant neoplasm affecting lymphoid tissue. Major lymph node groups will be affected in this condition. What are the major lymph node groups in the body? Are any of them normally palpable? Which are palpable when enlarged? What routine investigation can one do to determine the size of the nonpalpable group?

3. A 65-year-old male smoker complaining of cough, blood in his sputum and change in his voice is diagnosed as having a bronchogenic carcinoma. To which lymph node groups might this tumour spread? How does one detect their involvement? Why does the patient have a change in his voice?

4. The superficial inguinal lymph nodes are arranged in two groups: a horizontal group along the inguinal ligament and a vertical group along the terminal part of the long saphenous vein. Often one group may enlarge on its own without affecting the other. Diseases of which parts of the body affect the horizontal group specifically and which parts the vertical group?

Answers on page 388

The Lymphatic System

A Clinical problems

1. Secondary carcinomatous infiltration of the cervical nodes is common. The primary tumour can be anywhere in the oral cavity, nasal cavity, paranasal sinuses, nasopharynx, oropharynx, piriform fossa, larynx, thyroid gland or upper part of the oesophagus. Malignant tumours can also spread to the cervical nodes from the breast, bronchi, stomach and testes.

2. The major lymph node groups are the cervical, axillary, mediastinal, abdominal (pre-aortic and para-aortic) and inguinal nodes. None of these is normally palpable. When affected by malignancy or infection (lymphadenitis) all except the mediastinal nodes will become palpable. Abdominal nodes, enlarged in malignancy, may be felt on deep palpation. Enlargement of the mediastinal nodes can be detected on a plain X-ray of the chest.

3. A tumour from the lung spreading through the lymphatics can affect the hilar and tracheobronchial lymph nodes. Enlargement of these nodes may be seen on plain X-ray of the chest. Enlargement of the tracheobronchial nodes widens the angle at the bifurcation of the trachea. These nodes lie at the tracheal bifurcation. Widening of the angle will make the carina less prominent and this can be seen at bronchoscopy. These lymph nodes can compress the left recurrent laryngeal nerve and produce a change in the voice.

4. The horizontal group drains the lower part of the anal canal, ischiorectal fossa, lower part of the vagina, external genitalia including the vulva, the skin of the gluteal region and that below the umbilicus. It does not drain the testes or the ovary. Malignancy from any of these regions, or infection such as an ischiorectal abscess, can spread into the horizontal group of nodes and make them palpable. The vertical group drains the superficial tissues of the lower limb, except the back and lateral part of the leg. Infection, or a tumour such as melanoma, can spread primarily into the vertical group of inguinal nodes.

The Lymphatic System

5. Removal of the spleen (splenectomy) is the treatment of choice in cases of ruptured spleen and in conditions such as thrombocytopaenic purpura. Which peritoneal ligaments will the surgeon have to ligate and cut before the spleen is removed? What structures are housed in these ligaments? What happens to the size of the spleen when the splenic artery is ligated? Which organ is most vulnerable to damage during splenectomy?

6. Congenital thymic aplasia is also associated with non-development of the parathyroid glands. Why? Where do these structures develop? How will this condition manifest itself?

The Lymphatic System

5. The spleen is attached to the gastrosplenic and lienorenal ligaments. The former contains the left gastroepiploic and the short gastric vessels, and the latter the terminal part of the splenic artery and vein and the tail of the pancreas. The tail of the pancreas touches the spleen, and care is needed to avoid damage to it during splenectomy.

6. Interference with the embryonic development of the third and fourth pharyngeal pouches results in congenital thymic aplasia associated with hypoparathyroidism. Clinically, patients show hypocalcaemia, often associated with tetany, due to parathyroid deficiency. Peripheral lymphocyte counts show an absence of T-lymphocytes as a result of thymic aplasia.